THE W.E.T. WORKOUT

The W.E.T.

Water Exercise Techniques to Help

Workout

You Tone Up and Slim Down, Aerobically

JANE KATZ, Ed.D.

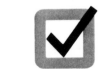

Facts On File Publications
New York, New York ● Oxford, England

The W.E.T. Workout
Water Exercise Techniques to Help You Tone Up and Slim Down, Aerobically

Copyright © 1985 by Jane Katz, Ed.D.

Library of Congress Cataloging in Publication Data

Katz, Jane.
  The w.e.t. workout.

  Includes index.
  1. Aquatic exercises. I. Title.
RA781.17.K38 1985   613.7'1   83-20829
ISBN 0-8160-0047-6 (HC)
ISBN 0-8160-0032-8 (PBK)

Printed in the United States of America

10 9 8 7 6 5 4 3 2 1

*This book is dedicated to
water lovers everywhere,
both the young
and the young at heart.*

Acknowledgments

I was inspired again to write a book about my favorite subjects, swimming and the wonderful world of water. Gladly, I'd like to offer special thanks to:

My parents—Dorothea and Leon, who introduced me to the wonders of water fun during infancy.

My sisters and brother—June Guzman, Paul Katz, and Elaine Kuperberg, for our time enjoying and playing in the water together.

Elaine Hochuli, M.A., Recreation Specialist—whose friendship, expertise and infectious enthusiasm has helped throughout.

My editor—Gerard Helferich, who has swum with me throughout.

My agent—Peter Skolnik, who has been most supportive out of the water.

Ann Jasperson—whose illustrations show the enjoyment of water exercise.

I'd also like to thank Howard Chislett, Ed.D., Herbert L. Erlanger, M.D., Margaret Johnson, Willibald Nagler, M.D., Marcelo Rodriquez, Mark B. Rosenman, Margaret Swan-Forbes, and the many sports medicine specialists who are most supportive of my W.E.T. Workout program, and the Facts On File staff members

Acknowledgments

who helped produce this book. And finally, thanks to all my student water lovers, from 6 months to 60 years and beyond, who have enjoyed W.E.T. Workouts.

Contents

Chapter 1

Take the Plunge

Water! It's the perfect environment for exercising, losing weight, toning up, and relaxing.

I'm going to show you how you can get the most out of exercising by following a conditioning program designed to be done in the water—exercises that I call "W.E.T. Workouts." They'll help you become fitter, better toned, more slender, and stronger.

Why is my W.E.T. Workout program better than any other exercise program? Simply put, water works! If you want to lose weight, get into shape, relax, feel sexy, or simply release the real "you" captured in a body suffering from too many extra pounds, too much stress, and too little exercise, my W.E.T. Workouts will work for you. This program will help you obtain the many benefits of exercise, enjoyably and without stress or pain.

Many types of exercises will help make you fit. Yet, let's face it, most of them aren't much fun. Most people don't enjoy sweating, straining, or pounding (and who can blame them?).

1

No one enjoys the risk of injury associated with jolting the body while jogging, or the strain of lifting weights or do calisthenic exercises designed by a contortionist.

However, I believe that exercising and suffering are not inseparable. You *can* enjoy yourself while becoming fit. And that's what my water exercise program is all about!

All exercise requires a certain amount of effort—but effort is different from discomfort. You can *enjoy* my W.E.T. Workout program while reaping its benefits. And if you enjoy doing something, you'll tend to stick with it.

My program includes W.E.T. Workouts for everyone—from challenging water exercises and techniques ("W.E.T.s") for the energetic, to relaxed programs for those who prefer a less vigorous routine. For those of you who are short on time, I've included exercises you can do during your lunch hour, without even getting your hair wet. For those of you with music in your soul, I've included exercises adapted from water ballet techniques. No matter what your taste, in *The W.E.T. Workout* you'll find an exercise program that will leave you refreshed, not fatigued; exhilarated, not exhausted. You'll improve your aerobic capacity, strength and flexibility; and the program will even help you lose weight!

Water, the "magic medium," is what makes my program different from—and better than—most other exercise regimens. For one thing, the medium itself is delightful. As soon as you get into the water, you feel relaxed as the day's tensions ebb away. Water is cool and delicious. It eases the mind as it strengthens the body; and it keeps you cool even if you exercise vigorously.

In the water your body feels almost weightless. The water supports you, adding grace and fluidity to your movements. This natural buoyancy allows your muscles, joints, and ligaments to move freely and comfortably, without pounding, straining, or jarring.

Water provides a natural resistance that helps tone and strengthen the muscles of your entire body. Your muscles have to work harder in water than in air, so you see the results of your exercise faster.

Water will help support, heal, and relax muscles that may be strained or tightened by other activities. If you have a sports injury, W.E.T. Workouts will help you recover quickly and return to your former level of fitness.

Finally, W.E.T. Workouts can be performed alone or in a group, and they can be done by swimmers and non-swimmers alike.

So, suit up and take the plunge into the exhilarating world of W.E.T. Workouts.

A Little Bit About Water

Water, water everywhere . . .

Most of the earth is composed of water. There's water surrounding us all the time. It's part of every living thing. Two-thirds of our bodies are made up of water. Many of our leisure pursuits take place in and around water (just check the travel section of any newspaper and note the photo suggestions). From earliest time, man has taken advantage of water's relaxing and healing properties. The Romans were famous for their baths, as are the Japanese. Popular natural mineral springs at Spa, Belgium added a new word to our language. In the 18th and 19th centuries, hydrotherapy, the use of water in the treatment of injury and illness, became very popular. Hydotherapists used cold water to reduce swelling caused by strains and sprains and to decrease fevers, and warm water was employed to increase blood circulation and to calm a patient. Many of the concepts of hydrotherapy are widely used today in modern physical therapy. For example, today physical therapists use underwater exercises to strengthen weakened muscles, to help relax torn and strained muscles, and to improve muscle function in patients recovering from strokes. Warm water massages (whirlpool tubs) are commonly used to help heal injuries and to promote relaxation.

Join the W.E.T. (Water Exercise Techniques) Set

In my program improve your aerobic fitness, increase your strength and flexibility, and ease the strain, tensions, and frustrations of everyday life—in water. I'll show you how to do this with a minimum of fuss. You can follow my program at any time of day.

A quick check of the Yellow Pages under "Health Clubs" will probably prove quite rewarding in finding facilities. Don't forget to check for local "Y's." You may also find that community centers and schools have pools open to the public; most large hotels and motels, and many smaller ones, having swimming facilities available to guests and to the public. Unless you're tripping off to the wilds, you should be able to find a place to do your W.E.T. Workouts—you can do them in lakes, ponds, and rivers, and on beaches. Don't let the weather put a damper on your program. In much of the world the summer is too short, so don't be afraid to do your swimming indoors for much of the year. And best yet, you can do W.E.T. Workouts privately if you're fortunate enough to have your own backyard pool, no matter what its size or shape.

Your biggest investment in W.E.T. Workouts, after access to a pool or other body of water, is a swimsuit. Swimsuits are

4

relatively cheap compared to other sports equipment. I recommend that women buy a "one size fits all" lycra suit, since these are very comfortable. Men can wear either a traditional boxer swimsuit or a nylon or lycra racing suit.

The W.E.T. exercises I describe can be used by everyone. No matter what your age or physical condition, this book offers you a program that will help you look and feel terrific. Since the program is progressive, you can get started without undue stress and strain, then gradually improve your level of fitness and maintain it. Each W.E.T. Workout will include a *warm-up*, a *main* or W.E.T. and a *stretch-out*.

Remember, it's never too late to start your W.E.T. progressive workout program. Improved aerobic capacity, flexibility, and strength are only the most obvious benefits you will derive from this program. Recent medical evidence has demonstrated that people who are physically fit are:

- able to keep their weight under control;
- sick less often;
- healthier in their outlook on life;
- less tense;
- younger looking;
- able to handle stress better.

So what are you waiting for?

Aerobics

What exactly are aerobic exercises? Those that benefit your cardiovascular system. No matter how big your biceps, without a strong cardiovascular system, you are not truly fit. Your cardiovascular system carries blood to your working muscles, supplying them with oxygen from the air you breathe and eliminating carbon dioxide and other waste products. Your ability to accomplish these biological tasks is commonly referred to as your "aerobic capacity." The stronger and more efficient your heart and lungs, the greater your aerobic capacity. The greater your aerobic capacity, the less strain on your heart, the greater your ability to perform work, the greater your ability to cope with stress, and the greater your feeling of well-being.

One of the most important goals in being physically fit is improving your aerobic capacity. There are other benefits to be gained from your W.E.T. Workouts, as well. These include improved endurance, greater coordination and strength, and an increased range of motion.

Safety Tips

Before beginning the W.E.T. program (or any other exercise program, for that matter) check with your doctor. This is especially important if you are not accustomed to regular exercise; if you are pregnant; if you are just a "weekend athlete"; if you are over 35 years of age; if you have recently recovered from an accident, injury, or illness; or if you suffer any physical condition, discomfort, or health problem.

Always listen to your doctor's advice, and never push yourself so hard that you experience pain or serious discomfort. Once you have a clean bill of health from your doctor, don't hesitate to get in the swim.

Good health—and most of all, have fun. Take the plunge!

Part I

W.E.T.s
(WATER EXERCISE
TECHNIQUES)

Chapter 2

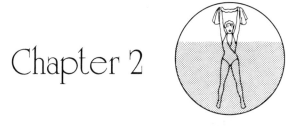

Introducing W.E.T.s

Here are your W.E.T.s (Water Exercise Techniques), which are the building blocks for all the W.E.T. Workouts in this book. They are organized into five groups—Warm-Ups and Stretch-Outs, Upper-Body, Middle-Body, Lower-Body, and Combination.

Warm-Ups and Stretch-Outs

Before each workout, you need to warm up; and after each water workout, you need to stretch out. Each warm-up and stretch-out session should last approximately five minutes. Warm-ups are essential because your body, especially the muscles, needs time to gear up, stretch, and get ready for action. If you don't warm up, you're more likely to strain a muscle or injure a joint. Stretching out after your workout helps you to relax, cool off, and bring your body back to its normal state.

Some of the warm-ups and stretch-outs I describe (e.g., bob-bing and breathing) will be standard exercises incorporated into most of the workouts. Remember that the best type of stretch is one that is slow and progressive—one in which you reach your maximum comfortable extension and hold for approximately 30 seconds. Remember that stretching should always be a slow and steady movement rather than a sharp and forced movement.

About Breathing

Throughout these exercises, breathe regularly, rhythmically, and deeply. Do not hold your breath. Remember to always inhale with your face out of the water, and to exhale with your face in the water, forming bubbles. Unless otherwise noted, inhale and exhale through both your nose and mouth.

Body Areas

The W.E.T.s in this section benefit the following body areas and muscle groups:

Upper Body

- head and neck (sternocleidomastoid)
- wrist, hand grip, and forearm (pronators)
- upper arm and back of arm (biceps and triceps)
- shoulders (deltoids)
- chest (pectorals)
- upper back (trapezius and latissimus dorsi)

Middle Body

- sides of trunk
- middle back
- rib cage (intercostals)
- waist (abdominals)
- lower back
- pelvic area

Lower Body

- thighs (hamstrings—back of thighs, quadriceps—front of thighs)
- groin, inner thigh (sartorius)
- buttocks (gluteus maximus)
- hips
- calves (soleus—front, gastrocnemius—back)
- knees
- ankle and foot (Achilles tendon)

Combination

Here, other W.E.T.s have been combined for total-body co-ordination. Create your own as you become more familiar with the program.

The W.E.T.s

For each W.E.T., I've provided a description of the starting position and of the technique, as well as an illustration. I've also given you a choice between a relaxed and a vigorous or energetic variation of each W.E.T. Depending on your needs, energy, time, and ability, you can choose the appropriate variation. It helps to know the standard technique before trying a variation.

Note that W.E.T.s can be combined to help you improve your coordination and utilize more muscle groups.

Getting Started: Gearing Up

Before you take the W.E.T. plunge, you'll need to gear up with just a few items.

Musts

SWIMSUIT

A stretch lycra or nylon suit is light, quick drying, and easily packed; plus, it is very comfortable.

My motto is don't leave home without it!: have suit, will travel (then you can do W.E.T. Workouts anywhere!).

PACE CLOCK OR WATERPROOF WRISTWATCH

Give each exercise and each workout session its full, allotted time. You will need a waterproof watch with a second hand or a pace clock (counting "1 Mississippi" gets boring) to keep tabs on the time. Don't cheat yourself.

Optionals (But Recommended)

SWIM CAP

If you're concerned about keeping your hair dry and protecting it, use a latex (rubber) cap.

If you prefer an easy-to-pull-on cap, or if you have long hair, a lycra (stretch) cap may be better. There are other new materials and caps available such as a silicone-base rubber cap.

GOGGLES

If you wear contact lenses or are sensitive to chemically treated water or salt water, you should use a pair of goggles. In addition to protecting your eyes, goggles allow you to see clearly underwater. It's a whole new universe!

Additional Equipment Suggestions

PULL-BUOY

A pull-buoy is a small, usually styrofoam, float often used by swimmers to support the lower body. A pull-buoy can be used both as a flotation device (placed behind the neck of a relaxed supine floater, or between the legs of a swimmer) and as a resistance device to be forced through the water during certain exercises.

KICKBOARD

A kickboard is a flotation device that supports the upper body, allowing swimmers to practice kicks. It also can be used as a resistance device.

FLOATS

These are inflated vinyl pouches that can be placed on the arms or legs. They can be used as a flotation device for easy, relaxed floating and/or as a resistance device.

FINS

Fins are large "paddles" that attach to the feet. There are many different weights, shapes, and styles. Commonly used for skin diving, they offer excellent propulsion and help to increase flexibility, strength, and speed. Use them for variations of lower leg W.E.T.s, i.e., in the medley of kicks.

HAND PADDLES

Paddles are resistance devices for the upper body. Placed on your hands, they offer greater resistance to the water (they're like fins for your hands). Try hand paddles when you perform upper-body W.E.T.s such as the medley of pulls.

WRIST AND ANKLE WEIGHTS

These are light, waterproof weights that can be used to increase water resistance during upper- and lower-body W.E.T.s. Try leg lifts with them, for example.

What to Look for in Water

Look for a swimming facility that is:

· Clean and safe
· Has a shallow area
· Has a comfortable water temperature (approximately 80° F)
· Has hours that fit into your lifestyle

Personal Safety Check

Check with your doctor before starting W.E.T.s, especially if you've recently been under a physician's care.

Listen to your body. If you experience any significant discomfort or pain, ease up on your exercises; if the problem persists, see your doctor.

Check the water depth and pool layout before you begin.
Be certain that your swimming facility is supervised properly (there should always be a lifeguard on duty).

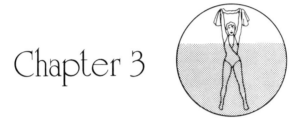

Chapter 3

Upper-Body W.E.T.s

ARM AND WRIST SWIRLS

Starting Position: Stand in shoulder-deep water. Extend your arms out from your sides and submerge them, bending your knees slightly.

Technique: Keeping your arms straight, rotate them in forward circles. Then vary with backward circles. Flex your wrists up and down as you rotate your arms.

For Variety

RELAXED: Create smaller, slower circles.

ENERGETIC: Create larger, more vigorous circles, using hand paddles for added resistance.

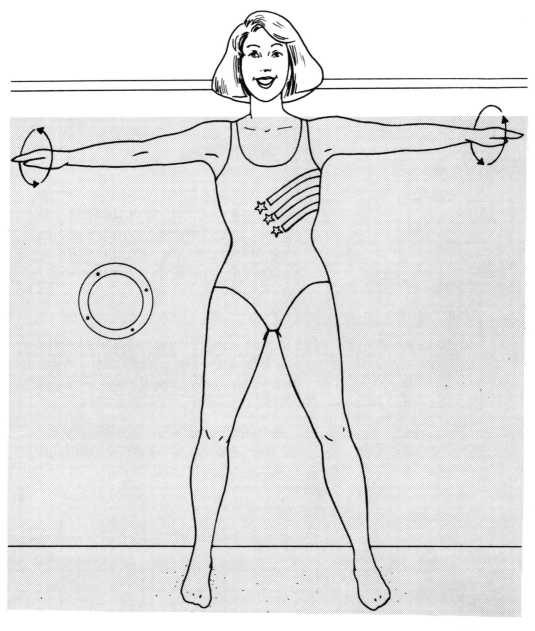

SPORT SWINGS AND FOLLOW-THROUGH

Special Benefits: Especially beneficial for tennis, paddle tennis, badminton, racquetball, squash, golf, baseball, bowling, and fencing; helps improve overhand swings, back-hand swings, forehand swings, and underhand swings.

Starting Position: Stand in chest-deep water; your arms out at your sides.

Technique: Move one arm forward, as if you were swinging a racquet. Follow through and recover out of the water, then swing your arm backward into the starting position. Repeat with the other arm.

For Variety

RELAXED: Practice a half-swing, stopping before you follow through. Keep your swing arm on the surface of the water to decrease resistance.

ENERGETIC: Use hand paddles or a pull-buoy for greater resistance. Follow through completely with each swing.

Tennis swing

Golf swing

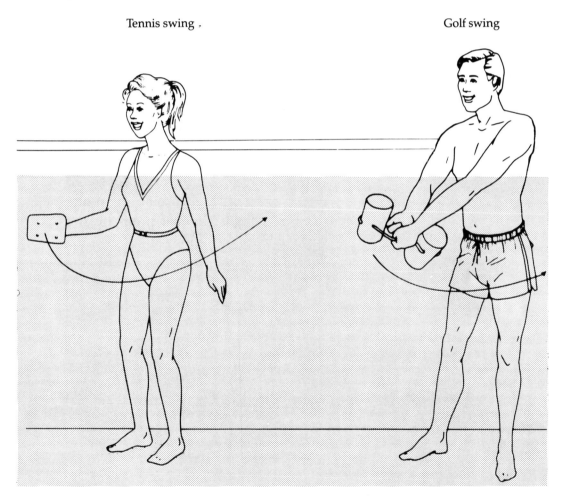

SPORT ARM PUMP

Special Benefits: Especially good for race walking, cross-country skiing, speed skating, boxer's punch, and fencer's parry.

Starting Position: Stand in chest-deep water with your feet shoulder-width apart.

Technique: With your fists closed, alternate your arms in a vigorous punching motion at shoulder level in front of you.

For Variety

RELAXED: Move your arms with a slower, longer follow-through, straightening your elbows fully on each arm extension.

ENERGETIC: Pump your arms more vigorously to create greater water turbulence; make the water "boil" by just breaking the surface with your elbows.

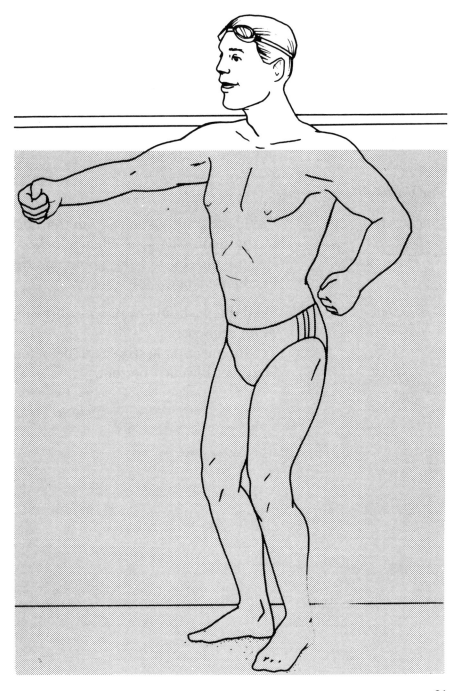

PUSH-UPS

Starting Position: Stand with your body facing the wall and touching it, your hands on the pool's edge, shoulder-width apart.

Technique: Straighten your elbows and lift your body out of the water.

For Variety

RELAXED: Stand an arm's distance from the side of the pool with your elbows locked. Bring your chest to the pool edge by bending elbows.

ENERGETIC: Hold the push-up position for three or more seconds.
Try the push-up in water too deep for your feet to touch bottom.

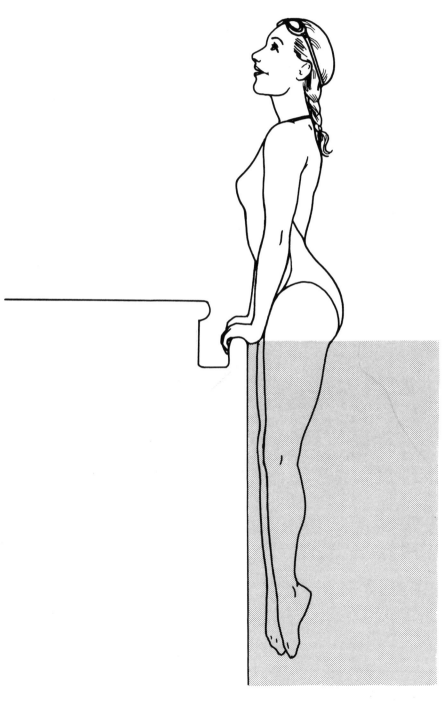

SCULL AND HUG

Special Benefit:	This is great practice for your sculling motion used in treading.
Starting Position:	Stand in chin-deep water, your arms extended in front of you with the thumbs pointing downward.
Technique:	Sweep your arms out and back as far as possible, pressing the water backward and keeping your thumbs down. Then turn your thumbs up and press the water forward, until your arms hug your body.

For Variety

RELAXED:	Turn your hands so that the palms face the pool bottom as you sweep your arms outward and forward. Bend your elbows as you sweep your arms.
ENERGETIC:	Use hand paddles for extra resistance, and to gain added flexibility try to touch your hands behind your back.

Starting position

Ending position

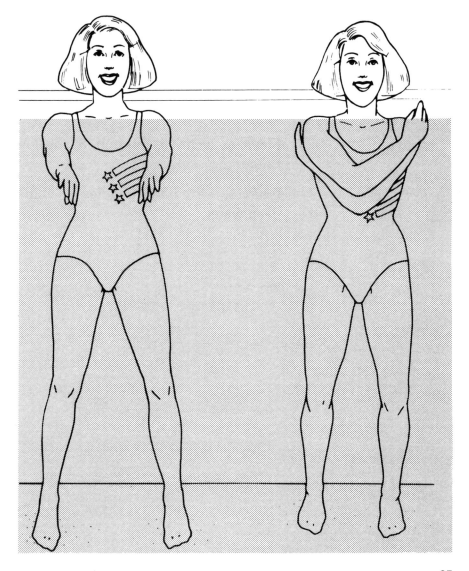

25

WATER PUSH

Starting Position: Stand in chest-deep water, your right arm extended behind you and your left arm stretched out in front of you.

Technique: With the palms facing down, press both arms toward the pool's bottom, then upward toward the surface in an underwater semicircle. Hold and repeat.

For Variety

RELAXED: Move your hand through a shorter range.

ENERGETIC: Exercise with hand paddles in chin-deep water.

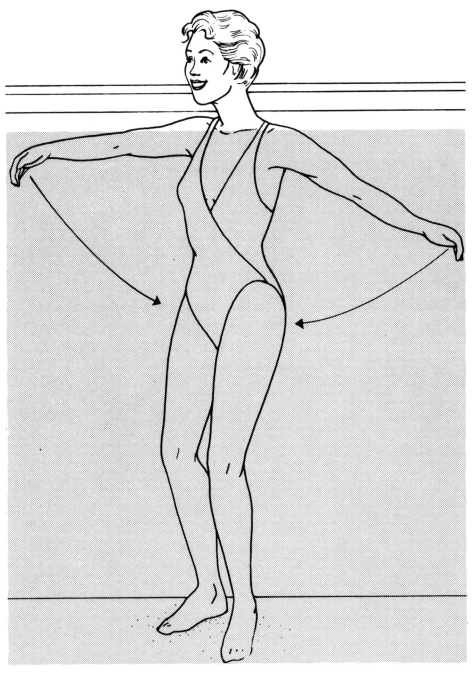

PULL-UPS

Technique:
With your back against the pool wall, in water of any depth, grasp the edge of the pool or a rung of the ladder, with your hands shoulder-width apart. Alternately pull your body up out of the water and slowly lower it back to a hanging position.

For Variety

RELAXED:
Start in a lower position and keep your arms slightly bent throughout the pull-up.

ENERGETIC:
Place your hands in a higher starting point (e.g., a diving board or starting block) and lift and lower your body as far as possible.

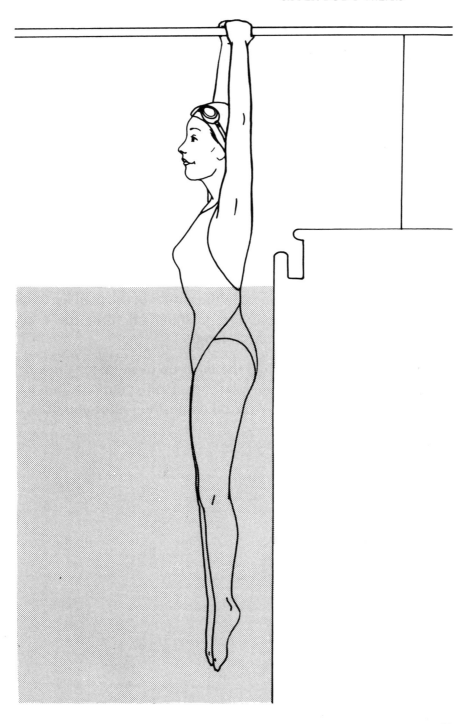

REAR PUSH-UP

Starting Position: Stand in waist-deep water with your back against the wall. Place your hands on the pool edge close to your sides, with your fingers pointing toward the water.

Technique: Straighten your elbows, lifting your body out of the water.

For Variety

RELAXED: Begin in the corner of the pool for easy leverage; pushing off from the pool bottom helps.

ENERGETIC: Hold the push-up position for three or more seconds. Bring your legs into an "L" or piked position after you lift.

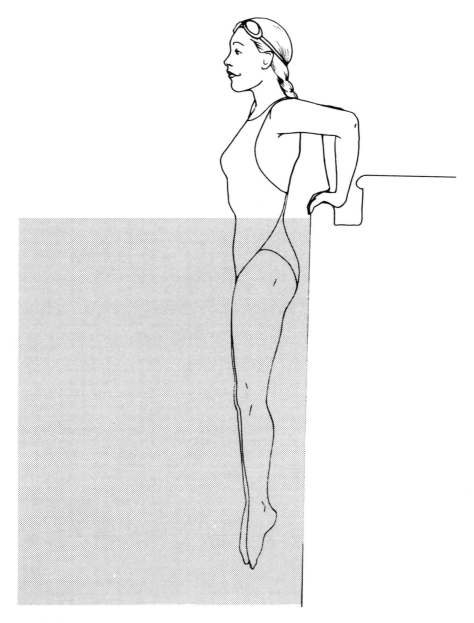

MEDLEY OF STROKES

Starting Position: Stand in shoulder-deep water.

Technique: Keeping your feet on the pool bottom, use the crawl stroke, breaststroke, or the sidestroke arm motion, or do a medley of all of these strokes.

For Variety

RELAXED: Stand in waist-deep water while practicing whatever stroke or strokes you wish.

ENERGETIC: Include the butterfly arm motion. Use hand paddles for additional resistance.

The crawl stroke

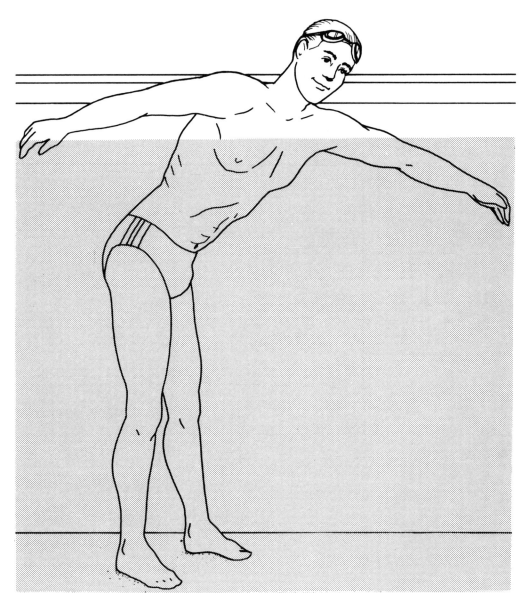

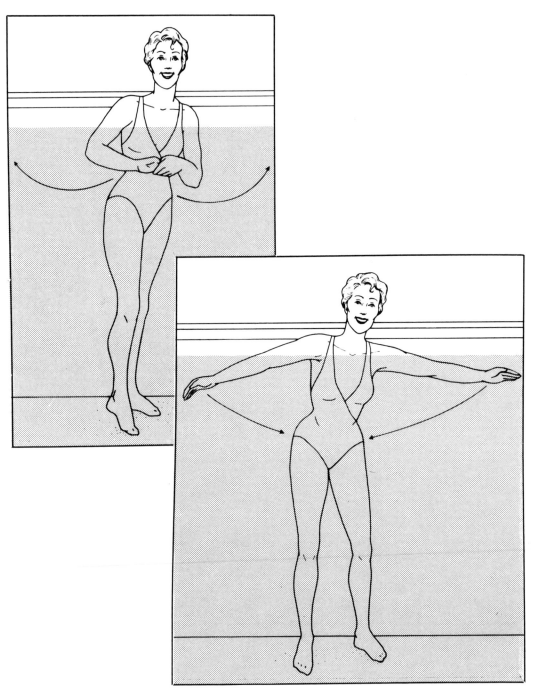

The sidestroke

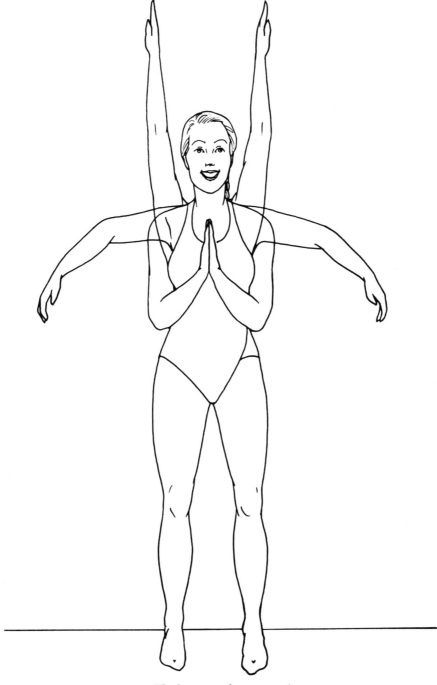

The breaststroke arm motion

REVERSE SCULL (SUPPORT SCULL)

Starting Position: Stand in chest-deep water. Bend your elbows 90° and hold them in front of you, your palms facing upward and your pinkie fingers together.

Technique: Move your palms out to your sides as far as possible while keeping your elbows touching your sides. Then move your forearms close together in front of your body again.

For Variety

RELAXED: Don't move your palms so far apart from each other—for example, only hip-width apart.

ENERGETIC: Cross your palms in front of you, pressing water upward to lower your body underwater.

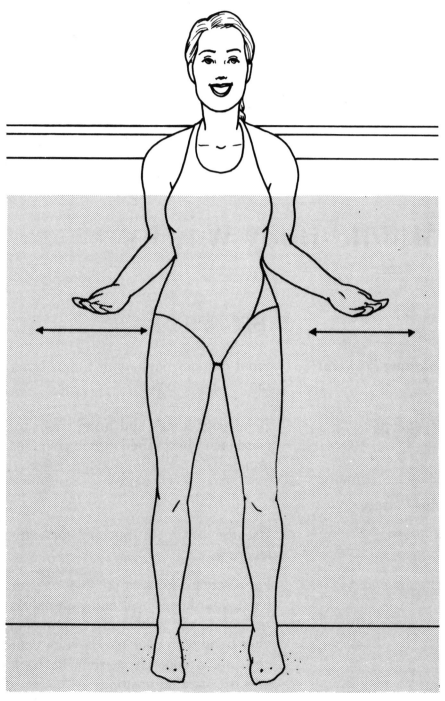

Chapter 4

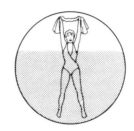

Middle-Body W.E.T.s

SIT-UPS

Starting Position:

Float on your back, your hands holding the pool's edge.

Technique:

Bend your knees and bring them toward your chest. Then extend your legs again.

For Variety

RELAXED:

Use the corner of the pool for extra leverage.

ENERGETIC:

For a very vigorous sit-up, float on your back, your knees bent and your calves resting on the pool deck. Supporting your head with your hands, tuck your chin up to your chest, then lie back into the starting position.

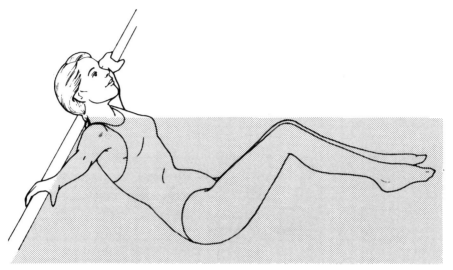

Relaxed position

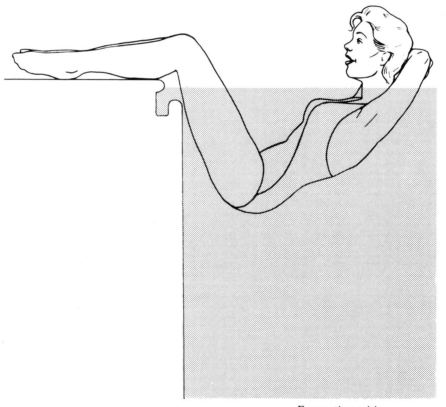

Energetic position

HIP TOUCH

Starting Position: Stand in chest-deep water, perpendic-
ular to the pool wall and one arm's
length from it.

Technique: Keeping your feet on the bottom, touch
your hip to the wall; then pull your hip
as far away from the wall as possible.
Repeat on the other side.

For Variety

RELAXED: Stand closer to the wall. Shift your
weight from one foot to the other,
rocking your hips from side to side.

ENERGETIC: Start farther from the wall.

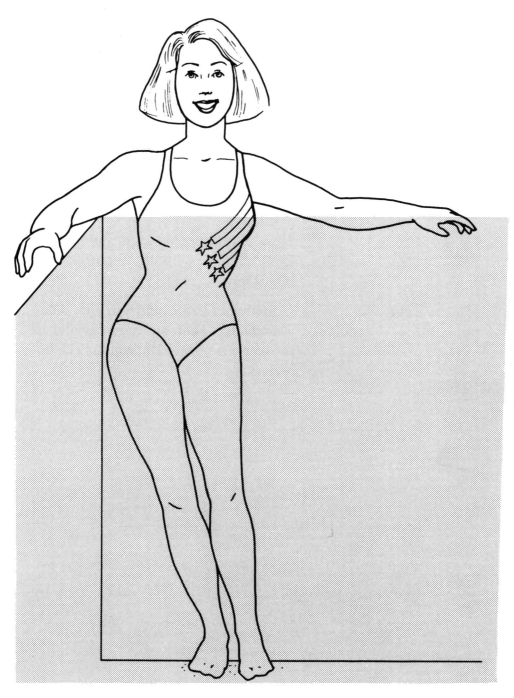

TRUNK TWIST

Starting Position: Stand in chest-deep water with hands on your hips.

Technique: Inhale as you twist your body to one side, then exhale as you return to the starting position. Repeat on the opposite side.

For Variety

RELAXED: Twist only your shoulders and head to each side without coordinating breathing.

ENERGETIC: Extend your arms out from your sides underwater, keeping them parallel to the water's surface throughout the exercise.

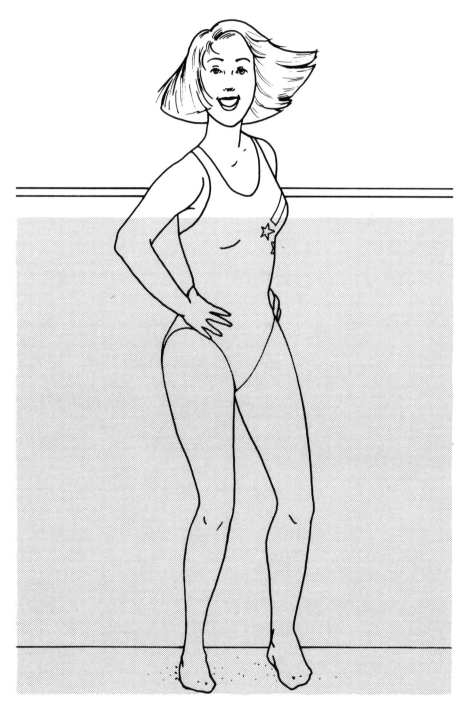

SPARE RIBS

Starting Position: Stand in waist-deep water with your feet shoulder-width apart. Extend your arms overhead.

Technique: Sway your arms overhead from side to side, feeling the stretch in your rib cage.

For Variety

RELAXED: Perform the sway with your hands behind your head.

ENERGETIC: Keeping your arms together, sway them in a counterclockwise circle across the front of your body, over the surface of the water and back to an overhead position. Change directions.

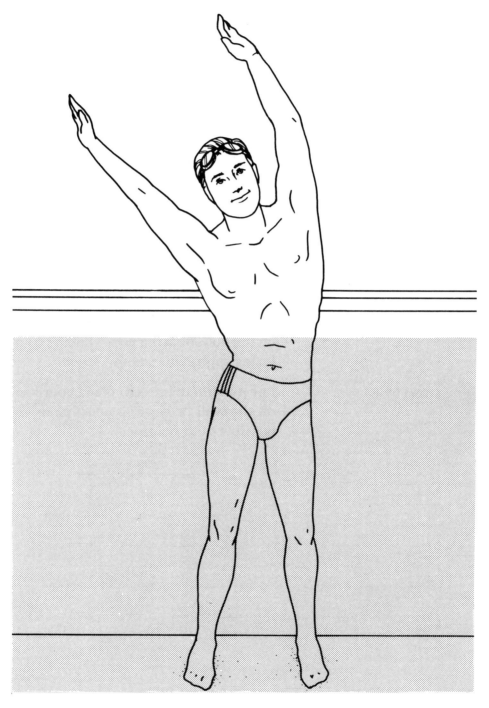

CRAB STRETCH

Starting Position: Position yourself with your back against the pool wall, corner, or ladder. Place the soles of your feet on the wall and hold onto the edge of the ladder with each hand.

Technique: Arch your back, straightening your legs as much as possible, with your head looking straight ahead. Slowly return to the starting position.

For Variety

RELAXED: For an easier stretch, keep your feet on the bottom of the pool, bending your knees slightly to feel the stretch.

ENERGETIC: For maximum stretch, place your feet on the wall as close to your hands as possible, and hold.

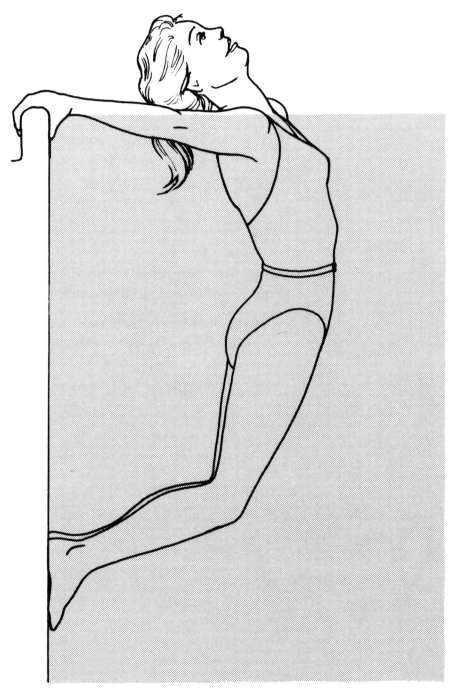

47

BUTTOCK SQUEEZE

Starting Position: Stand with your back in a corner of the pool, one hand on either edge and your elbows bent.

Technique: Press your hips forward and tighten your buttocks. Then relax your buttocks and allow your hips to return close to the wall, and repeat.

For Variety

RELAXED: Squeeze your buttocks together without pressing your hips forward.

ENERGETIC: Add a pelvic tilt to the buttock squeeze and bring your body to a back float position.

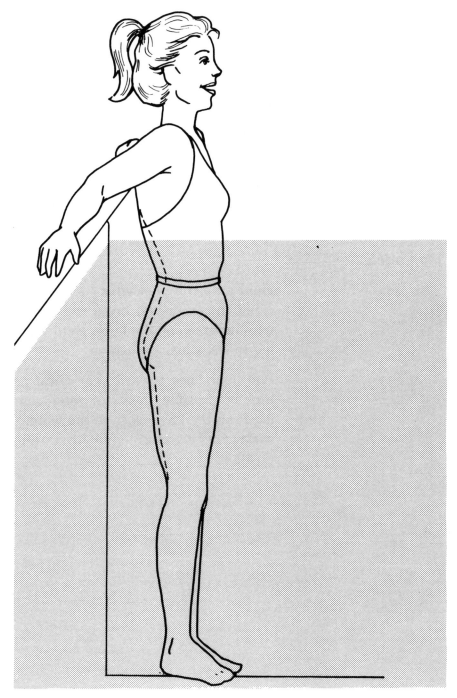

KNEE TUCK

Starting Position: Stand in chest-deep water, with your back against the wall.

Technique: Grasp one knee and bring it toward your chest. Then release your leg and extend it forward by straightening the knee. Return the leg to the starting position.

For Variety

RELAXED: Hold onto the pool edge for support. Bend the knee and bring the leg up without grasping the knee. Return the leg to the starting position.

ENERGETIC: Pull your knee toward your chest as high as possible, then straighten your leg from the knee close to the water's surface before returning to the starting position.

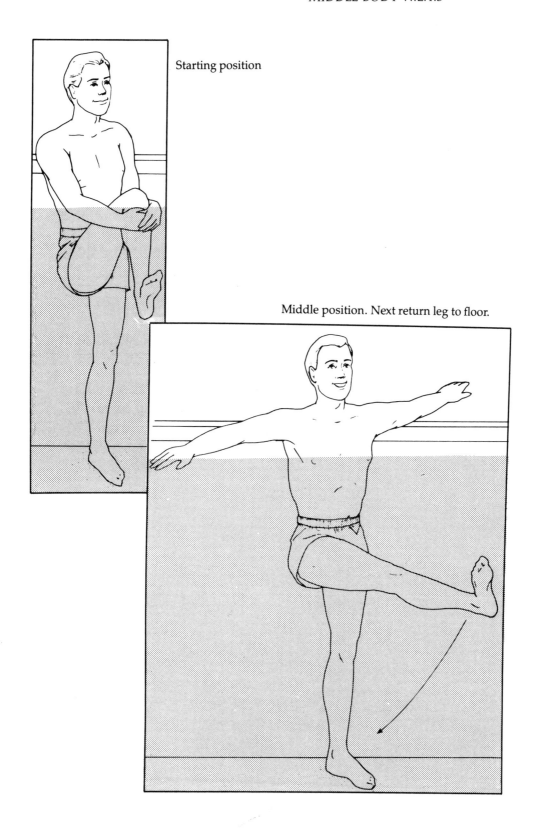

Starting position

Middle position. Next return leg to floor.

LEG SWING

Starting Position: Stand with your back to the corner of the pool in any depth of water, one hand on either edge and with your arms slightly bent.

Technique: Pike at the waist by lifting your legs, creating an "L" with your body. Maintain the "L" as you twist your body and swing your legs first to the right, then to the left.

For Variety

RELAXED: Bend your knees as you swing your legs.

ENERGETIC: Extend your arms for a wider starting position. Twist your body in an "L" shape and swing your legs from right to left, touching your toes to each wall.

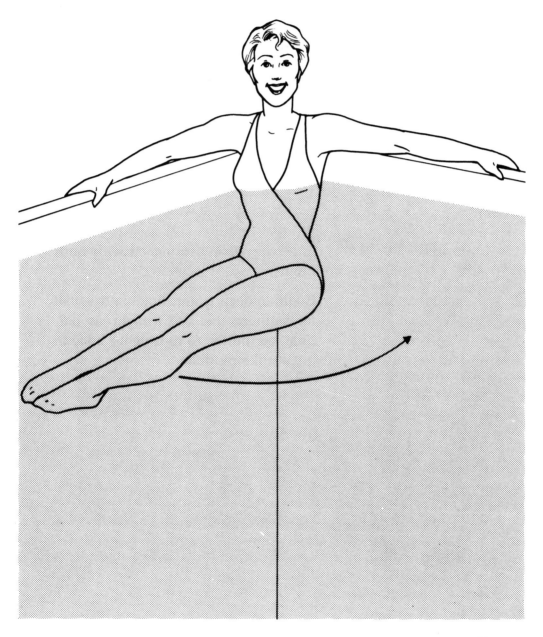

BODY WAVE

Starting Position: Stand close to the wall in chin-deep water, holding onto the wall with one hand.

Technique: With legs together, press your hips alternately forward and backward, keeping your knees relaxed and allowing your hips and legs to perform a sinuous, wavelike motion.

For Variety

RELAXED: Face the wall, holding on with both hands.

ENERGETIC: Begin in deep water, holding the wall for support, and use a vigorous dolphin leg motion to move your body in a wavelike motion.

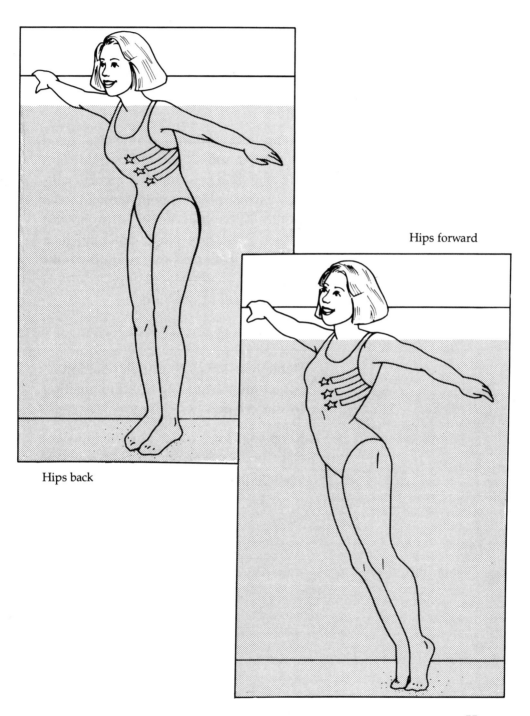

Hips forward

Hips back

PENDULUM SWITCH

Starting Position: Begin in a back float position with your arms at your sides.

Technique: Using your abdominal muscles, bend your hips and slowly lower them into the water. Then reach forward with your arms, placing your face into the water. Keep your knees straight and extend your legs back, finishing in a prone float. Reverse by rounding your back and bending your hips to return to a back float position.

For Variety

RELAXED: Bend your knees to a tuck position as you change from one floating position to the other.

ENERGETIC: Keep your form as streamlined as possible, and squeeze your buttocks as you change position.

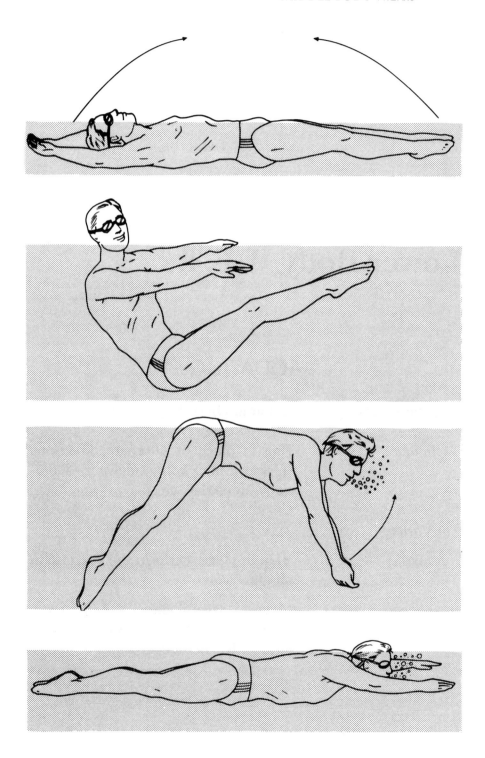

Chapter 5

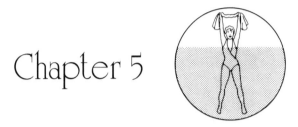

Lower-Body W.E.T.s

AQUA-JOG

Starting Position: Begin in chest-deep water.

Technique: Run in place or alternate directions (forward, backward, sideways, diagonally, in circles, etc.).

For Variety

    RELAXED: Skip in place. Perform the exercise in shallow water.

    ENERGETIC: Move in several directions—forward, backward, sideways—taking longer strides. Run in deeper water.

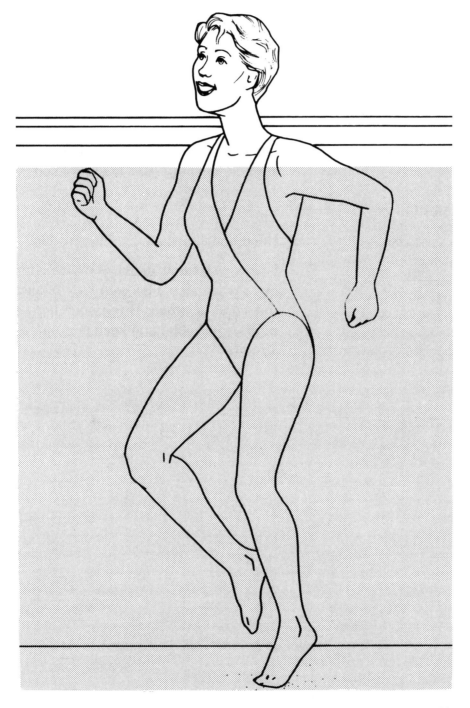

ROCKETTE KICK

Starting Position: Stand in chest-deep water, your back against the pool wall. Hold onto the pool edge for support.

Technique: Lift one leg at a time to the water's surface, keeping your knees locked.

For Variety

RELAXED: Bend your knee as you lift your leg.

ENERGETIC: Use a pull-buoy under your heel for extra resistance. Flex your foot to keep the buoy in place. Bring your leg as high as possible, and keep your knees straight.

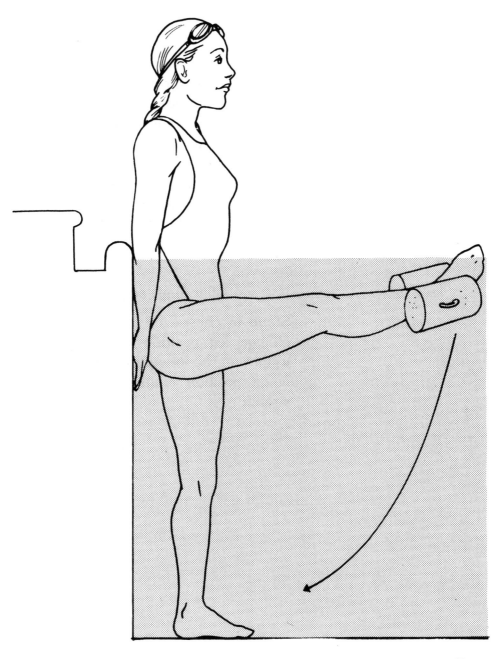

LEG LUNGE

Starting Position: Stand in waist-deep water.

Technique: Take one large lunge-step forward with your right foot, the right knee bent and the left leg straight. Press your body weight through your hips to feel the stretch on the inner thigh. This exercise can also be done by stepping sideways (as in a fencing lunge) as far as possible. Return to a standing position and repeat on the other side.

For Variety

RELAXED: Use a smaller lunge step.

ENERGETIC: Stand in chest-deep water. Jump to change leg positions, keeping your weight on the forward leg. Hold each lunge position longer for an extra stretch.

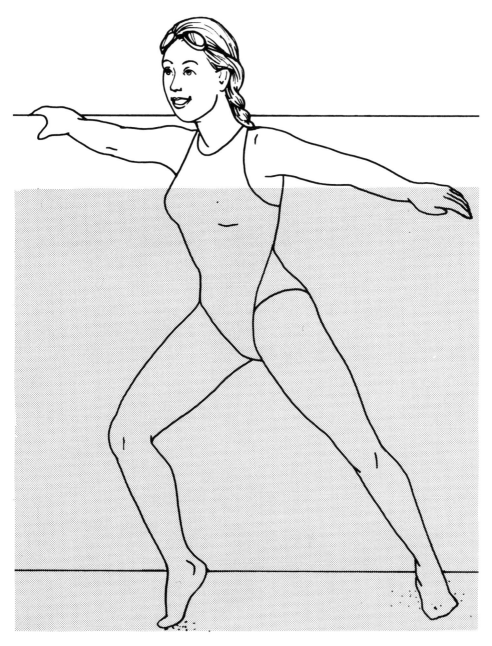

PLEA SQUEEZE

Starting Position: Stand in waist-deep water, holding onto the edge of the pool for balance. Touch your heels together and turn your toes outward.

Technique: Make a deep-knee bend (plea), then squeeze your buttocks together as you straighten up. Keep your hips in line with your shoulders throughout.

For Variety

RELAXED: Squeeze your buttocks, bending your knees only slightly.

ENERGETIC: Repeat the plea squeeze with your feet shoulder-width apart. (Ballet lovers, do the plea squeeze in all six ballet positions.)

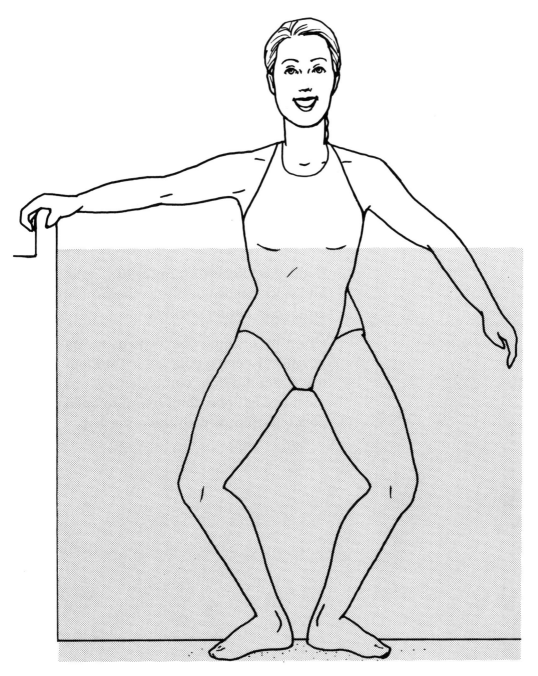

LEG CROSSOVER

Starting Position: Put your arms over the sides of the pool and place your back against the wall. Lift your legs to a 90° angle, keeping them straight and together.

Technique: Separate your legs into a "V", then bring them back together. Alternately open and close your legs. Maintain the "L" shape, and keep your legs straight.

For Variety

RELAXED: Bend your knee to form a 90° angle, and place one leg over the other, knees crossed in sitting position.

ENERGETIC: Begin by opening your legs as far as possible. Keeping your left leg stationary, bring the right completely over to meet the left one, then return to open position. Repeat with the other leg.

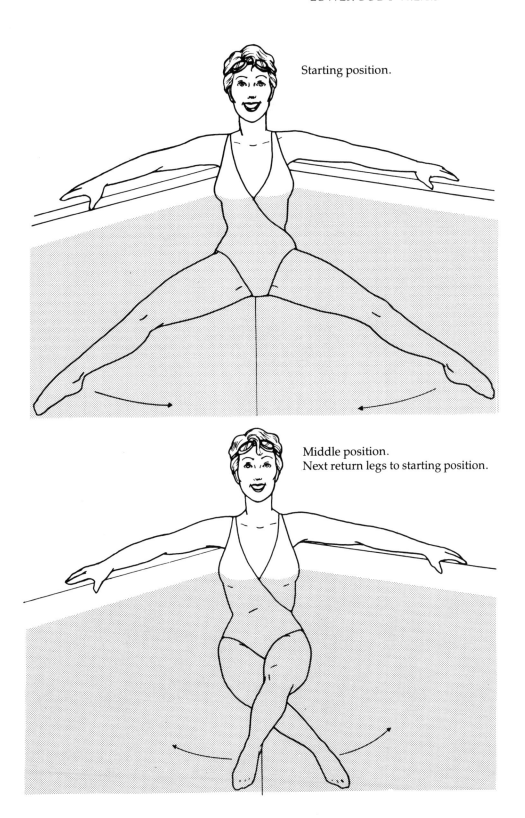

Starting position.

Middle position.
Next return legs to starting position.

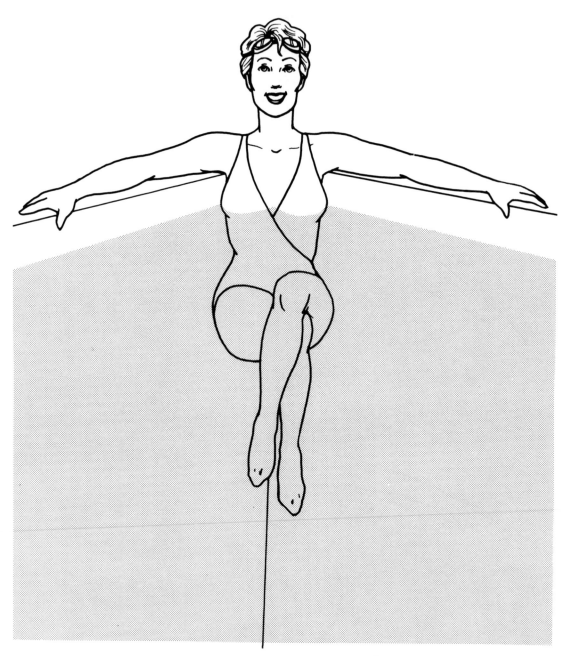

Leg Crossover, relaxed position

DISCO AQUA DANCER

Starting Position: Stand in chest-deep water, your feet together.

Technique: Bend your knees and move your body from side to side in a step-together-step dance sequence.

For Variety

RELAXED: Try the slower dance steps—e.g., fox-trot, waltz, etc.

ENERGETIC: Try the more vigorous dance steps, e.g., square dances. Point and flex your feet in square-dance style (keeping your hands up under your chest).

69

SIDE SWIPE

Starting Position: Rest your arms and hands lightly on the deck and stand with your back against the wall at the corner.

Technique: Alternately bring one leg out to the side, then down and across your standing leg toward the opposite wall in a semicircular pattern.

For Variety

RELAXED: Move your leg in a smaller circle, bending the knee if necessary.

ENERGETIC: For extra resistance, place your heel between the floats of a pull-buoy. Try the exercise without holding onto the wall.

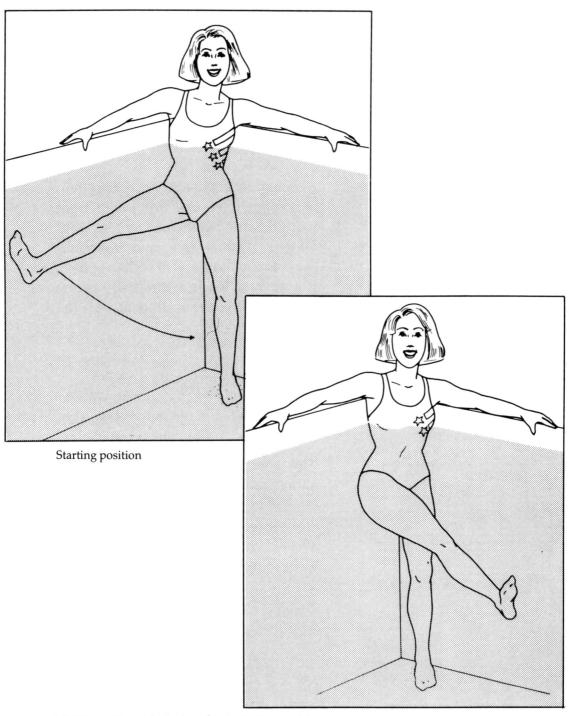

Starting position

Middle position. Next return leg to starting position.

KARATE KICK

Starting Position: Stand in chin-deep water at the corner of the pool, your back to the corner and your arms fully extended out away from your sides. Hold onto the pool sides for support.

Technique: Keeping your knees close together, bend your knee and bring your right foot up behind you close to your right buttock. Then rotate your knee outward and touch the wall with your heel. Rotate your leg in a circle to resume the starting position. Repeat with the left leg.

For Variety

RELAXED: Support your body by placing your elbows on the side of the pool, so that the distance to the wall is reduced.

ENERGETIC: Kick your legs vigorously in an alternating motion, one leg following the other. Move away from the corner, releasing your hands from the wall, keeping your body out of the water and as high as possible.

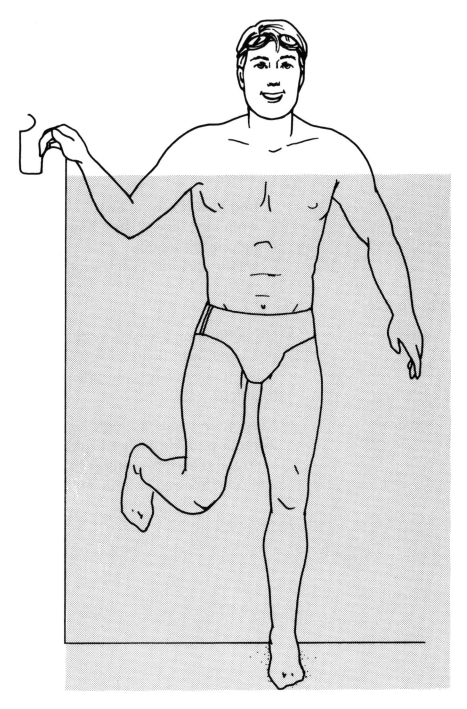

LEG TREADING

Starting Position: Begin in chin-deep water, one hand resting lightly on the pool edge, a safety line, or a buoy.

Technique: Use one or more of the following leg motions:

- frog kick (knees apart)
- whip kick (knees close together)
- bicycle leg motion
- scissor kick (as in sidestroke)

For Variety

RELAXED: Use a flotation device (i.e., kickboard, pull-buoy, arm float) to support your upper body while you practice leg treading.

ENERGETIC: Keep your hands as high out of the water as possible while treading. (This leg tread is used by water polo players and synchronized swimmers.)

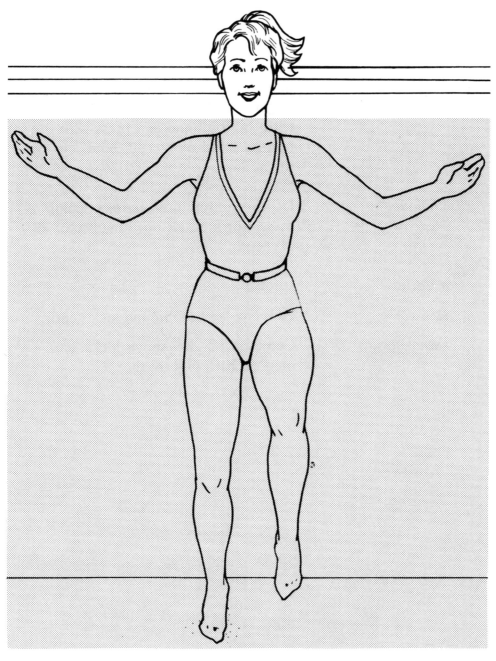

MEDLEY OF KICKS

Starting Position: Face the pool wall and assume the bracket position: i.e., hold onto the edge with one hand and press the other hand against the wall under the water, fingers pointing downward. Then pull with the top hand and press with the bottom hand as you lift your legs to the surface.

Technique: Do the flutter, breaststroke, dolphin or scissor kick, or do a medley of all of them.

For Variety

RELAXED: Pick one leg motion and kick gently.

ENERGETIC: Combine all the above kicks into a medley. Kick vigorously.

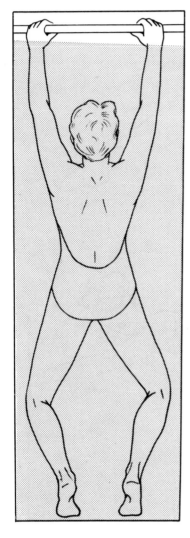

Breaststroke kick

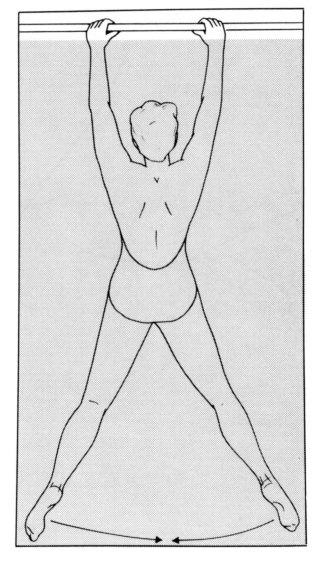

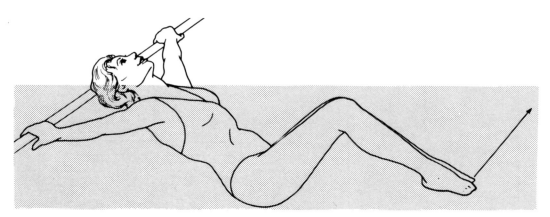

Supine dolphin kick

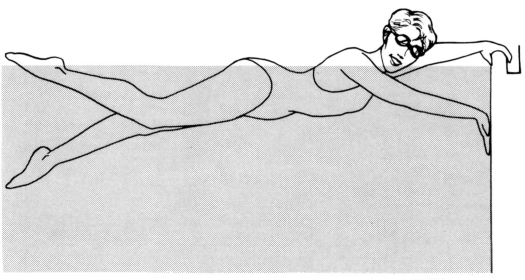

Flutter kick

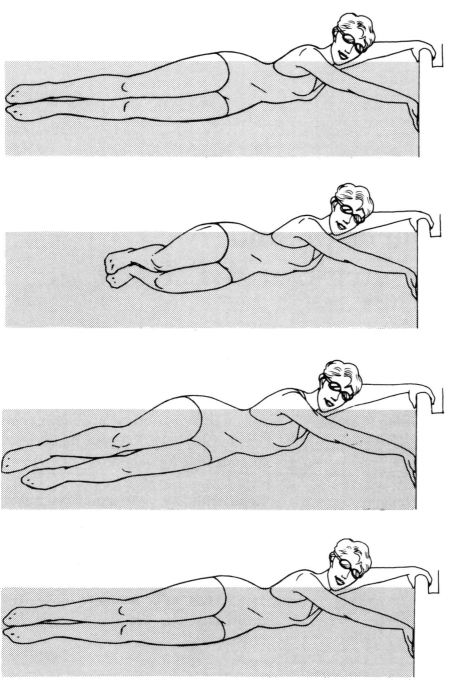

Scissor kick

79

Chapter 6

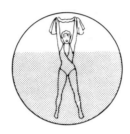

Warm-Up and Stretch-Out W.E.T.s

TOE TESTER

Starting Position: Sit on the edge of the pool with your legs in the water. Put your hands next to your hips for support.

Technique: Begin with foot circles: move your feet inward, downward, outward, and upward in a circular motion. With your knees slightly bent, use an alternating up-and-down leg movement (flutter kick), keeping your ankles loose. Try a breaststroke kick and some leg crossovers.

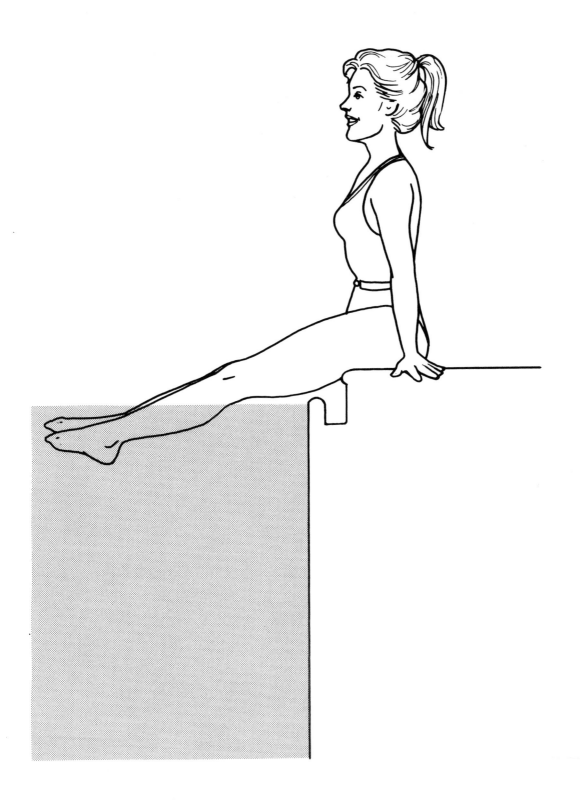

BREATHING AND BOBBING

Starting Position: Stand in chest-deep water.

Technique: Bend your knees slightly until your chin is at water level, then exhale so that you create ripples in the water in front of you. Submerge and exhale underwater, forming bubbles. In both phases, inhale through your nose and mouth and exhale completely through your nose and mouth.

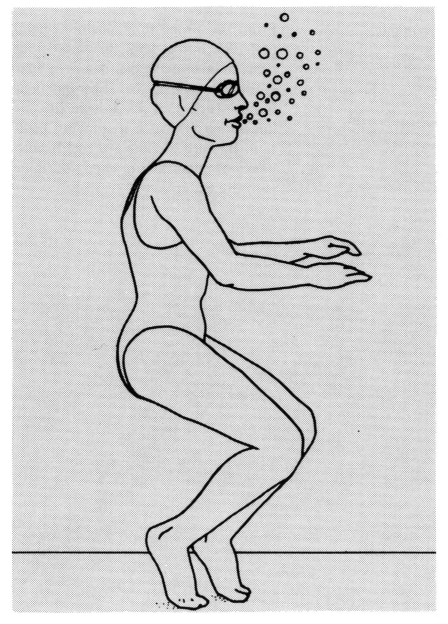

FETAL FLOAT

Starting Position: Begin in a prone position (face down).

Technique: From the prone float position, bend and tuck into a fetal (jellyfish) float position by bringing your knees to your chest and grasping your shins with your hands. Tuck your head down to your knees and return to a standing position. Be sure to exhale through both your nose and mouth when your face is in the water.

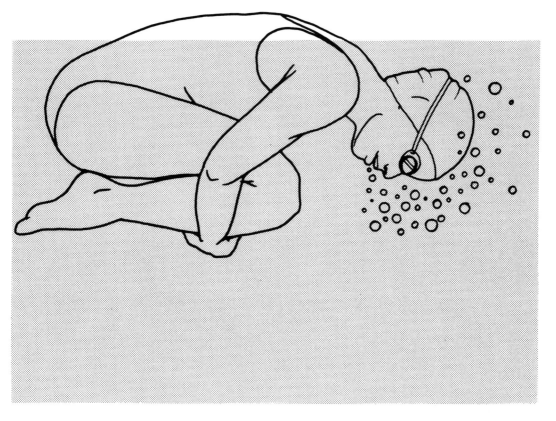

BACK ARCH STRETCH

Starting Position: Standing in shallow water, face the pool wall and place your hands on the deck or a rung of the ladder so that your lower body is in an arched push-up position.

Technique: While holding onto the deck, gradually bring your hips, body, and head out of the arched position and into a rounded position by straightening your elbows.

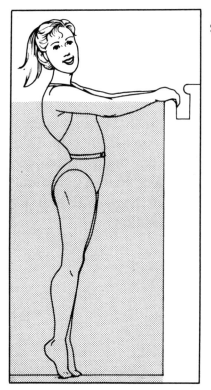

Starting position

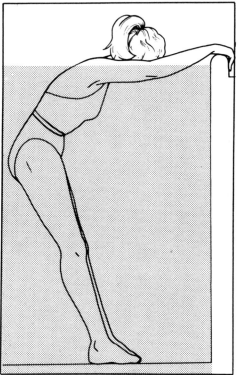

Ending position

STANDING TALL

Starting Position: Standing in shoulder-deep water, place your back against the pool wall.

Technique: Press your back, head, shoulders, buttocks, and heels against the wall. Take one step away from the wall, keeping your posture perfect. Return to the wall by taking a step backward and rechecking your position.

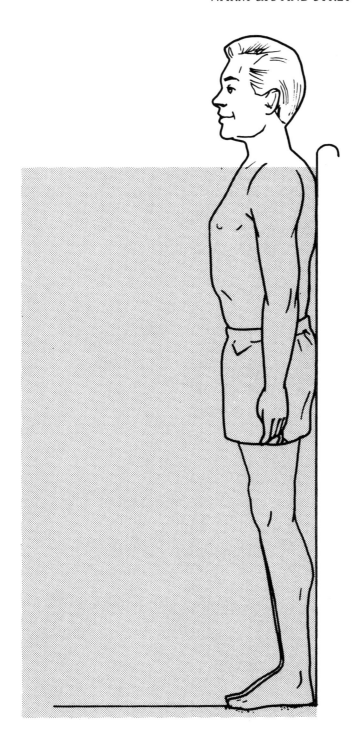

STATIC ARM STRETCH

Starting Position: In chest-deep water stand next to the pool wall with one hand on the wall.

Technique: Slowly stretch by pressing one shoulder forward toward the wall and hold for 30 seconds. Change arms and repeat.

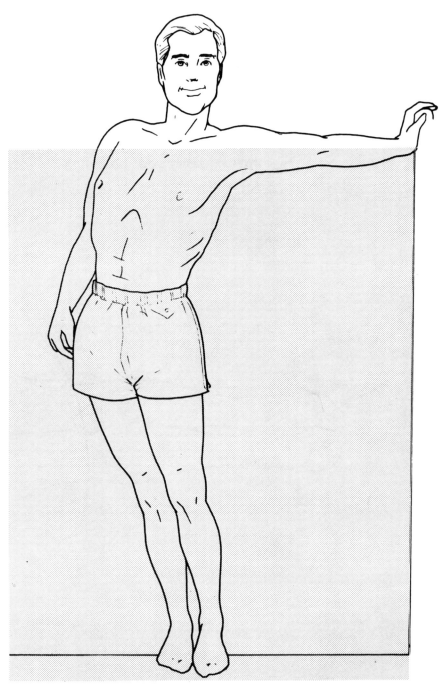

LOG ROLL

Starting Position: Begin by floating horizontally.

Technique: Keeping your arms at your sides, rotate your body by turning your head and shoulders in one direction. Experiment and let your body flow.

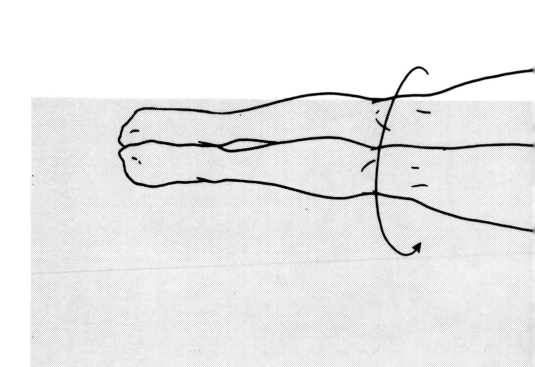

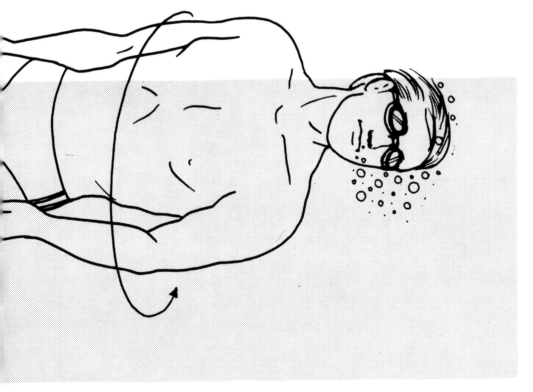

PIKE BODY STRETCH

Starting Position: Facing the wall, hold onto the pool edge with both your hands; bend your knees and place your toes against the wall below your hands.

Technique: Slowly extend your legs and arms into a piked position and hold it. Place your heels flat against the wall. Gradually return to starting position.

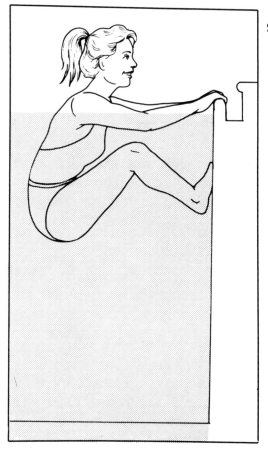

Starting position

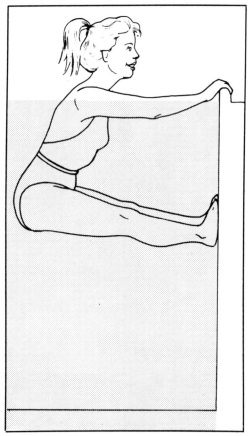

Ending position

LEG SPLIT

Starting Position: Stand facing the pool wall in waist-deep water, both hands on the edge; turn out your feet and place them where the wall and bottom meet.

Technique: To increase your split, press upward with your hands as you extend your legs to a split position.

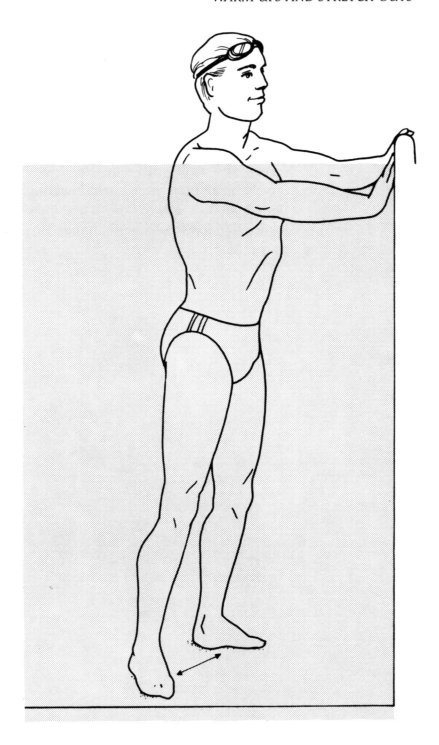

STATIC BALLET LEG STRETCH

Starting Position: Standing in waist-deep water parallel to the pool wall, place one foot on the edge.

Technique: Grasp the wall with one hand and slowly straighten your knee, lowering your body as close to your leg as possible. Hold for 30 seconds. Change legs and repeat.

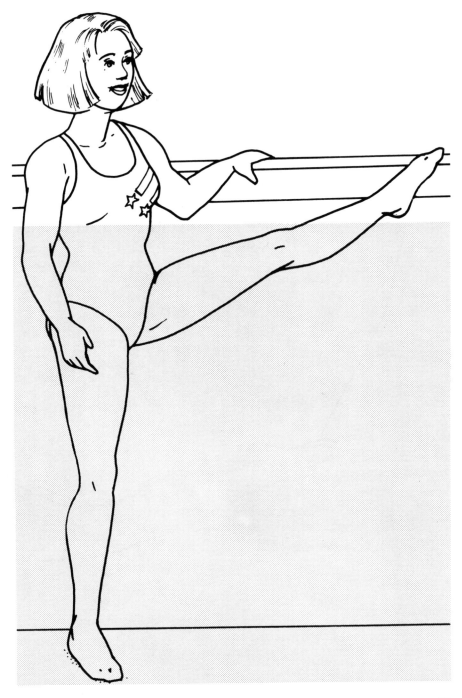

UPWARD BOUND

Starting Position: Begin in a prone float position.

Technique: Let your body relax and bend slightly forward at the waist. Take a breath by pressing your hands downward and outward in a wide sculling motion to lift your head out of the water. Then place your face in the water and exhale. Repeat this breathing continuously.

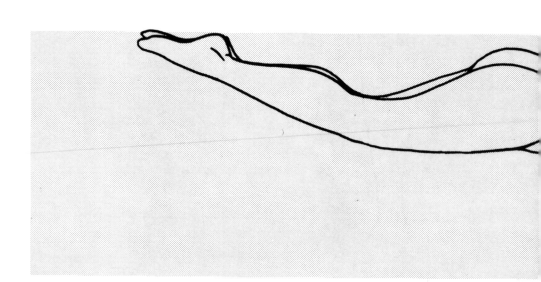

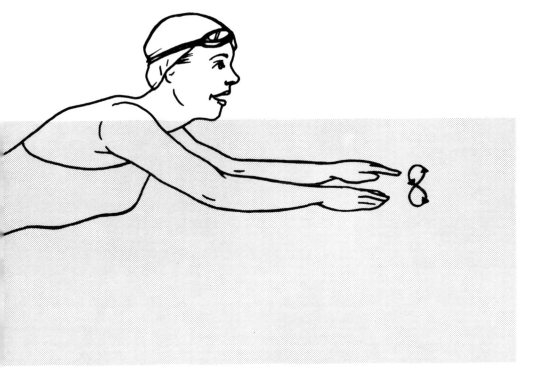

RUNNER'S LEG STRETCHES

Starting Position:

Stand in chest-deep water, parallel to the pool wall, with one arm extended and your hand on the deck.

Technique:

First, move your right foot backward and stretch the leg's calf muscle by touching your heel to the pool's bottom. Repeat with the other foot.

Follow this by bending your right leg behind you, heel toward the buttock, and grasping your right foot with your right hand to pull your foot upward, stretching your thigh muscle. Hold for a count of five. Lower your foot and repeat with the left leg.

Starting position   Ending position

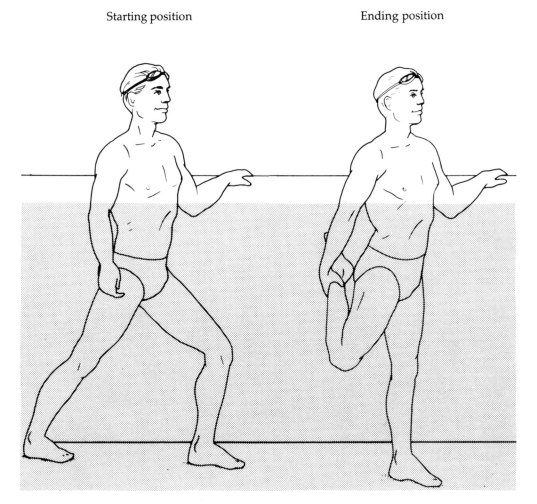

HEAD CIRCLES

Starting Position: Stand in neck-deep water, your hands at your sides.

Technique: Slowly rotate your head in a clockwise, then counterclockwise, motion. Lift your head forward, then lower it backward.

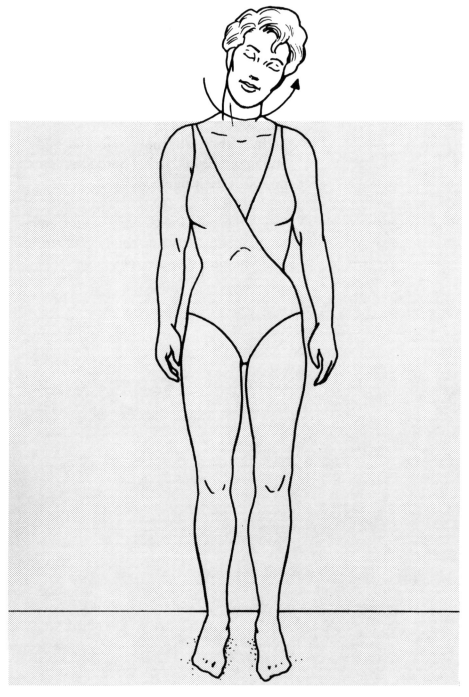

SHOULDER SHRUG

Starting Position: Stand in shoulder-deep water, your arms at your sides.

Technique: Lift your shoulders up and down together; then alternate left and right shoulder shrugs. Bring both shoulders forward, then backward.

For Variety: Try "chicken wings." Place your hands on your shoulders and rotate your arms and shoulders in a circle.

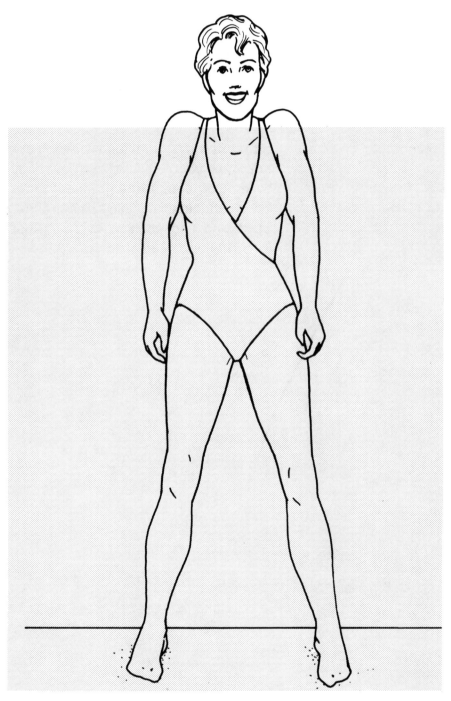

OVERHEAD STRETCH

Starting Position: With both hands, grasp either end of a wand, stick, or rolled-up towel. Place it behind your neck.

Technique: Either in water or on land, extend your arms over your head. Stretch your body by moving your arms gradually from left to right, keeping your arms straight. Start and end each W.E.T. workout with this overhead stretch.

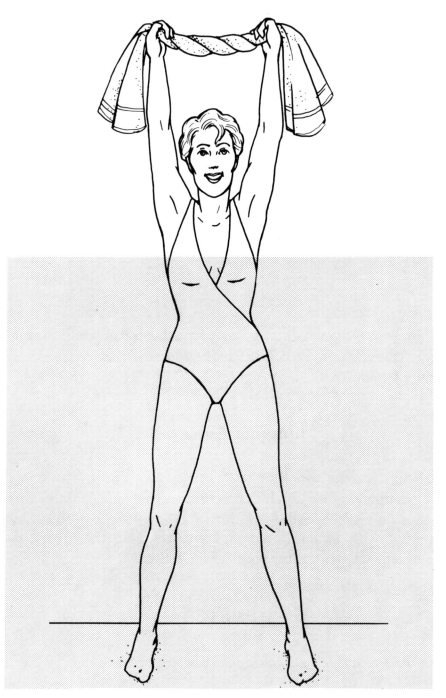

Chapter 7

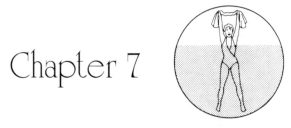

Combination W.E.T.s

Some of the preceding W.E.T.s have been combined to provide combination W.E.T.s. Create your own as you become more familiar with the program.

Jumping Aqua Jack

Begin by either standing or floating on your back. Turn your palms upward and touch them overhead as you separate your legs into a "V" position. Return to the starting position by turning your palms downward and bringing them back to your sides as you bring your legs together.

Ballet V

An arm and leg stretch-out. Standing in chest-deep water, grasp your right inside heel with your right hand and slowly

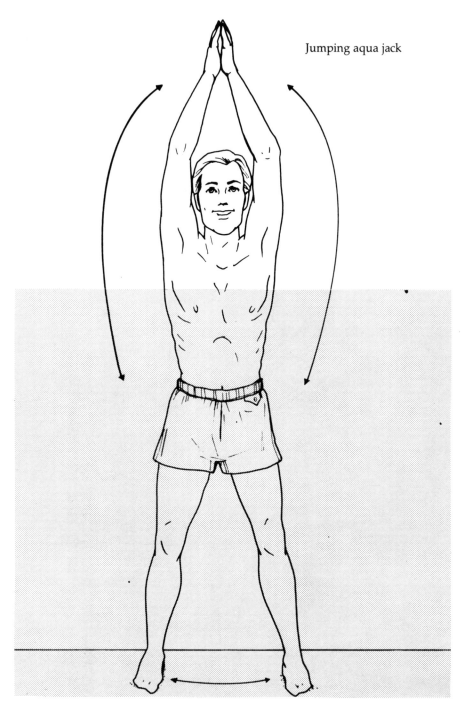

Jumping aqua jack

straighten your knees while balancing on your left. Return to starting position by bending both arms and legs simultaneously.

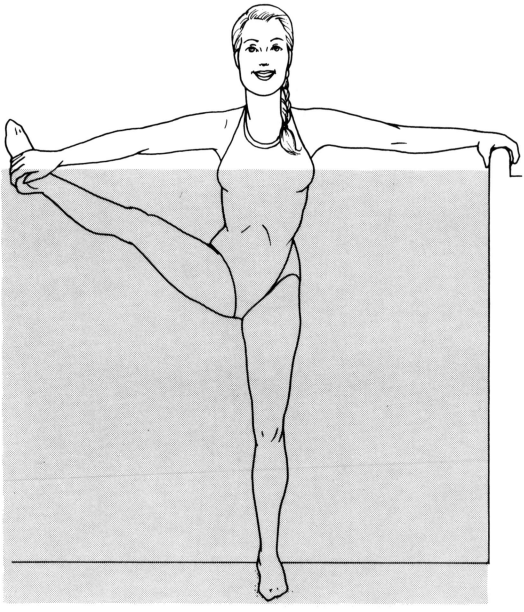

Ballet V

Crossover Toe Touch

Standing in chest-deep water, lift your right Rockette leg and tap your left hand to your right foot. Alternate with your right hand touching your left foot.

Coordinated Sport Arm and Leg Motions (Your Choice)

Practice your favorite sport motion, coordinating arm and leg action. Example: Take a step forward as you make a forehand tennis swing. Or jump rope, ski, ride a horse, etc.

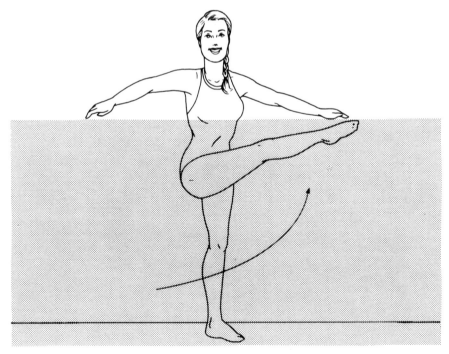

Crossover toe touch

The Freestyler

Begin in chest-deep water for all strokes. As you do an aqua jog, use the crawl stroke arm motion; add rhythmic breathing by turning your head to one side as your opposite arm is extended.

W.E.T. Workouts mean different strokes for different folks. Coordinate the arm motions of the following strokes in chest-deep water.

- *The Backstroker*

  As you aqua jog backward, use backstroke arm motion.

The backstroker

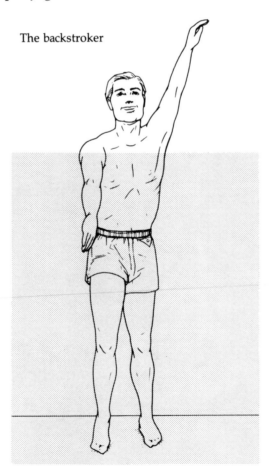

- *The Breaststroker*

  With forward aqua jog or jump use a breaststroke arm motion. Keep arms underwater for the outward scull motion and recovery. Add your breathing by lifting head at the start your pull.

- *The Sidestroker*

  With a sideways aqua jog, pull and press arms using a sidestroke arm motion.

- *The Butterflyer*

  With forward aqua jog use butterfly arm motion by creating large forward arm circles together.

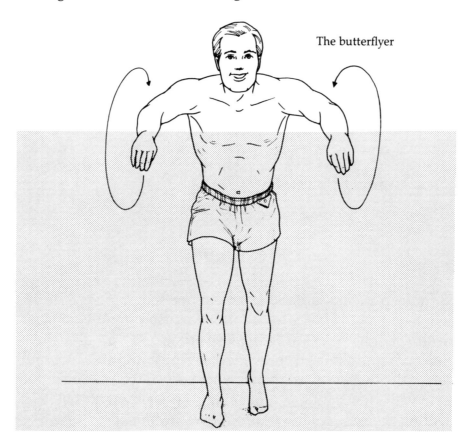

The butterflyer

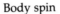

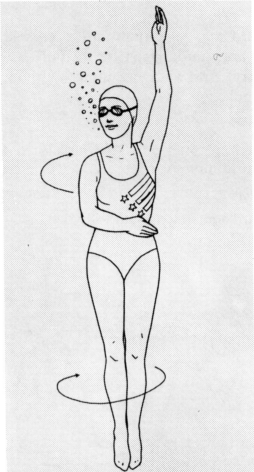

Body Spin

In deep water, submerge at least one foot in a vertical position with both your arms extended outward from your sides at shoulder level, palms facing forward in a "T" position. Spin your body to the right by vigorously pushing water to your left with your right arm moving across your chest. Finish the spin with your right hand touching your waist on the left side. During the spin, your left arm moves overhead.

Treading

In treading, you use the arms and legs to maintain a vertical position in deep water with little energy. Begin in a sitting position, with your shoulders over your knees, in chin-deep water. The arms perform a wide sculling motion, while the legs can use any of the following motions: a bicycle leg motion, scissor kick, frog kick, whip kick, or eggbeater motion.

Tug-of-War

In chin-deep water, use a reverse scull as you tread with your legs. The scull will press you underwater while the treading will keep you up. See which is *your* better half!

Tug-of-war

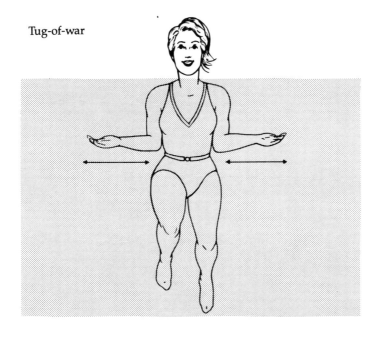

Invent Your Own Stroke

Combine different leg motions with different arm motions (e.g., from a back float position, use backward arm circles [butterfly arms] with a frog kick [breaststroke leg motion]).

Part II

THE PROGRESSIVE 12-WEEK W.E.T. WORKOUT PROGRAM

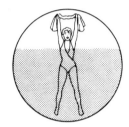

Chapter 8

Introducing the W.E.T. Workout Program

Now you're suited up and ready to take the plunge for your first W.E.T. Workout, the beginning of the progressive 12-week program I've designed to optimize your total fitness. Why 12 weeks? Because three months is a realistic period of time for getting into shape. In these 12 weeks you'll be able to develop a weekly routine of doing W.E.T.s. I recommend that you do your W.E.T.s 3 times per week (every other day is best). However, if your schedule won't accommodate this, do the best you can. You'll benefit from doing your W.E.T.s even once a week.

The following chart outlines your level of fitness from week 1 to week 12 and beyond.

W.E.T. Workout Components

All the suggested W.E.T.s (Water Exercise Techniques) that make up each workout are described in the preceding W.E.T. section. Each W.E.T. Workout contains the following components:

WARM-UP

W.E.T. SET

SHAKE OUT

STRETCH-OUT

Warm-Up

As I've already noted, the warm-up is an important part of your workout. *Don't skip it!* It gets you moving, it gets the blood flowing, and it prepares your body for the W.E.T. set. It also prepares your joints and muscles to move more easily through their full range of motion. Your warm-up should also include a comfortable adjustment to the water (bobbing is a great technique for this).

W.E.T. Set

This is the "meat and potatoes" portion of your workout. Each main set includes W.E.T.s for each body area—upper, middle, lower—as well as exercises to improve your coordination. As you become more fit, your W.E.T. set will increase in duration from 10 minutes to 20 minutes and more. Arrange the exercises as you desire, but be sure you do the exercises for each body part. To help you remember your main W.E.T. set, jot it down on a 3 × 5 card and place it at poolside. In each W.E.T. set, there are optional relaxed and energetic segments. Let your preference, energy, time, and ability dictate

122

how you will exercise. As you progress, challenge yourself to the more energetic variations.

To help determine your energy output, check your pulse. This will help you keep a check on your cardiovascular progress. First, take your resting heart rate (RHR): While you're relaxed, place your index finger on either side of your neck or the inside of your wrist; take your pulse for six seconds and add a zero. This will give you your resting heart rate. Your RHR will be most accurate in the morning when you're rested and relaxed (but before you have a cup of coffee).

To determine your theoretical maximum heart rate (MHR), use the American Heart Association's formula: MHR = 220 − Age.

When doing your W.E.T. set, try to keep your heart rate at your target heart rate, which is about 75% of your maximum heart rate.

To estimate your Target Heart Rate (THR), take your pulse for 6 seconds immediately after your W.E.T. set. Don't wait too long because your pulse rate drops off quickly after exercise. Remember your 6-second THR pulse count is only "a ball park figure." However, if it's way too high or too low, adjust your pace to bring your pulse to the THR.

Shake Out

As part of your W.E.T. set, do a "shake out" between segments for each body part. The shake out is a rest period to help re-energize, loosen, and relax your muscles before you begin the next part of the W.E.T. set. Think of the shake out as a *shimmy*. Bob up and down, relax, and shake your arms and legs. Take up to a minute for each "shake out." If you feel fatigued, rest for short intervals of approximately 30 seconds to 1 minute between each W.E.T.; but avoid getting chilled.

Stretch-Out

The stretch-out segment of your workout helps your body to slow down and relax, gradually bringing your heart rate and breathing back to your normal resting rate. The stretch-out should last about 5 minutes.

How to Improve Your F.I.T.ness With Your 12-Week Progressive W.E.T. Workout Program

1st Month (Weeks 1-4)

Take the plunge. Get geared up, get set, and go for it—a lifetime of fun and fitness awaits you!

In the first month, your main W.E.T. set should last approximately 10 minutes. Each exercise is performed for 1 minute. Remember your 5-minute warm-up and 5-minute stretch-out, for a total 20-minute water workout.

2nd Month (Weeks 5-8)

Get into shape! Your main W.E.T. set increases by 5 minutes and is now approximately 15 minutes in length. Try the optional swim equipment, and check your pulse.

3rd Month (Weeks 9-12)

You're on your way to becoming aerobically fit! Your main

W.E.T. set increases by 5 minutes, becoming 20 minutes in length. Try new workout variations.

Week 13 and Forever After

Stay in shape and maintain your new level of F.I.T.ness. You can have more fun by varying your W.E.T. Workouts.
As you become more F.I.T., try:

Frequency	• Increasing the number of workouts per week.
	• Increasing the number of repetitions per exercise.
	• Increasing the number of W.E.T.s per workout.
Intensity	• Increasing the intensity of your W.E.T.s with fins, hand paddles, etc.
	• Increasing the difficulty of your W.E.T.s, from relaxed to energetic.
Time	• Increasing the length of your main set, up to 40 minutes.
	• Substitute rest periods for shake-outs between W.E.T.s.
	• Increasing or varying the length of time devoted to each W.E.T.

Remember at all times to enjoy yourself as your F.I.T.ness increases. Be energized rather than enervated.

Be creative. Combine various W.E.T.s to suit your interests. Other W.E.T. Workout variations are described in the following section. These include water activities in spas, family and partner games, beach and open-water activities, and more.

Now gear up and take the plunge!

Chapter 9

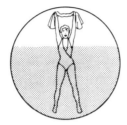

The Workouts

W.E.T. PROGRESSIVE WORKOUT

Week 1

You've taken the plunge and are off to a great start. Try to do your W.E.T. Workout every other day.

Warm-Up
(5 min.)

Toe Tester
Breathing and Bobbing
Standing Tall

W.E.T. Set
(10 min.)
1 minute
per exercise

Upper: Water Push
Push-ups

SHAKE OUT

Middle: Trunk Twist
Sit-ups

SHAKE OUT

Lower: Aqua-jog
Side Swipe

SHAKE OUT

Combination: The Freestyler

Stretch-Out
(5 min.)

Static Arm Stretch
Runner's Leg Stretches
Upward Bound

W.E.T. PROGRESSIVE WORKOUT

Week 2

You may be experiencing some muscle soreness. Don't worry, your body will become adjusted to your W.E.T. program. Stay with it!

WARM-UP
(5 min.)

Overhead Stretch
Breathing and Bobbing
Leg Split

W.E.T. SET
(10 min.)

Upper: Arm and Wrist Swirls
      Rear Push-up

SHAKE OUT

Middle: Body Wave
      Pendulum Switch

SHAKE OUT

Lower: Medley of Kicks
      Leg Lunge

SHAKE OUT

Combination: Treading

STRETCH-OUT
(5 min.)

Shoulder Shrug
Back Arch Stretch
Static Ballet Leg Stretch

W.E.T. PROGRESSIVE WORKOUT
Week 3

Use the W.E.T. sport skills you like and know for the combination.

WARM-UP (5 min.)	**Toe Tester** **Breathing and Bobbing** **Head Circles**
W.E.T. SET (10 min.)	**Upper: "Scull and Hug"** 　　**Sport Swings and Follow-Through**
	SHAKE OUT
	Middle: Buttock Squeeze w/Crab Stretch 　　**Spare Ribs**
	SHAKE OUT
	Lower: Karate Kick 　　**Disco Aqua Dancer**
	SHAKE OUT
	Combination: Coordinated Sport Arm 　　　　**and Leg Motions** 　　　　**Ballet V**
STRETCH-OUT (5 min.)	**Runner's Leg Stretches** **Leg Split** **Upward Bound**

W.E.T. PROGRESSIVE WORKOUT

Week 4

Hidden fitness: What you see is not all you get! Your W.E.T. workouts are designed to improve your aerobic capacity too!

WARM-UP
(5 min.)

Toe Tester
Upward Bound
Back Arch Stretch

W.E.T. SET
(10 min.)

Upper: Medley of Strokes
    Sport Arm Pump

SHAKE OUT

Middle: Hip Touch
    Crab Stretch

SHAKE OUT

Lower: Leg Crossover
    Plea Squeeze

SHAKE OUT

Combination: The Breaststroker
    Crossover Toe Touch

STRETCH-OUT
(5 min.)

Breathing and Bobbing
Log Roll
Standing Tall

W.E.T. PROGRESSIVE WORKOUT
Week 5

Congratulations! After 4 weeks, you're getting into shape with your W.E.T. Workouts. Your bonus is 5 minutes added to your main set. You're ready!

WARM-UP
(5 min.)

Breathing and Bobbing
Leg Split
Shoulder Shrug

W.E.T. SET
(15 min.)
(add 5 minutes)

Upper: Push-ups
      Reverse Scull
      Sport Arm Pump

SHAKE OUT

Middle: Sit-ups
      Pendulum Switch
      Trunk Twist

SHAKE OUT

Lower: Rockette Kick
      Side Swipe
      Aqua-jog

SHAKE OUT

Combination: The Backstroker
      Treading with Tug-of-War

STRETCH-OUT
(5 min.)

Head Circles
Upward Bound
Overhead Stretch

W.E.T. PROGRESSIVE WORKOUT
Week 6

Do this W.E.T. Workout with swim equipment for variation: e.g., fins (for legs), hand paddles (for arms) or arm floats (for upper body).

WARM-UP (5 min.)	**Toe Tester** **Log Roll** **Leg Split**
W.E.T. SET (15 min.)	**Upper: Scull and Hug** **Water Push** **Medley of Strokes**
	SHAKE OUT
	Middle: Spare Ribs **Buttock Squeeze** **with Crab Stretch** **Body Wave**
	SHAKE OUT
	Lower: Medley of Kicks **Rockette Kick** **Side Swipe**
	SHAKE OUT
	Combination: Jumping Aqua Jack **The Freestyler**
STRETCH-OUT (5 min.)	**Static Arm Stretch** **Static Ballet Leg Stretch** **Upward Bound**

W.E.T. PROGRESSIVE WORKOUT
Week 7

Try some new upper-body techniques and The Butterflyer. Don't forget to check your pulse.

WARM-UP (5 min.)	**Runner's Leg Stretches** **Shoulder Shrug** **Back Arch Stretch**
W.E.T. SET (15 min.)	**Upper: Pull-ups** 　　　**Arm & Wrist Swirls** 　　　**Reverse Scull**
	SHAKE OUT
	Middle: Hip Touch 　　　**Leg Swing** 　　　**Knee Tuck**
	SHAKE OUT
	Lower: Leg Treading 　　　**Plea Squeeze** 　　　**Leg Lunge**
	SHAKE OUT
	Combination: The Butterflyer 　　　**Crossover Toe Touch**
STRETCH-OUT (5 min.)	**Log Roll** **Leg Split** **Pike Body Stretch**

W.E.T. PROGRESSIVE WORKOUT
Week 8

You're W.E.T. Workout now has 3 combination exercises. Keep up the great work!

Warm-Up
(5 min.)
	Breathing and Bobbing
	   Pike Body Stretch
	   Static Arm Stretch

W.E.T. Set
(15 min.)
	Upper: Rear Push-up
	   Sport Arm Pump
	   Medley of Strokes

SHAKE OUT

Middle: Crab Stretch
   Sit-ups
   Body Wave

SHAKE OUT

Lower: Leg Crossover
   Karate Kick
   Disco Aqua Dancer

SHAKE OUT

Combination: The Side Stroker
   Jumping Aqua Jack
   Crab Stretch

Stretch-Out (5 min.)	**Standing Tall** **Upward Bound** **Overhead**

W.E.T. PROGRESSIVE WORKOUT
Week 9

Now that you're in shape, your W.E.T. set increases to 20 minutes. Let's do each W.E.T. for 1½ minutes.

Warm-Up (5 min.)	**Toe Tester** **Head Circles** **Shoulder Shrug** **with "Chicken Wings"**

W.E.T. Set (20 min.) 1½ minutes per exercise	**Upper: Pull-ups** **Sport Swings and Follow-Through** **"Scull and Hug"** SHAKE OUT **Middle: Pendulum Switch** **Spare Ribs** **Knee Tuck** SHAKE OUT **Lower: Plea Squeeze** **Rockette Kick** **Leg Treading** SHAKE OUT **Combination: The Backstroker** **Body Spin** **Ballet V**

Stretch-Out (5 min.)	**Leg Split** **Pike Body Stretch** **Upward Bound**

W.E.T. PROGRESSIVE WORKOUT
Week 10

For a new W.E.T. Workout variation, use a crescendo interval: 1 minute, 1½ minutes, then 2 minutes for each body part.

WARM-UP (5 min.)	**Breathing and Bobbing** **Back Arch Stretch** **Static Ballet Leg Stretch**	
W.E.T. SET (20 min.)	**Upper: Push-ups**	(1 min.)
	Medley of Strokes	(1½ min.)
	Water Push	(2 min.)
	SHAKE OUT	
	Middle: Leg Swing	(1 min.)
	Sit-ups	(1½ min.)
	Buttock Squeeze with Crab Stretch	(2 min.)
	SHAKE OUT	
	Lower: Karate Kick	(1 min.)
	Medley of Kicks	(1½ min.)
	Aqua-jog	(2 min.)
	SHAKE OUT	
	Combination: The Butterflyer	(1 min.)
	Treading	(1½ min.)
	Jumping Aqua Jack	(2 min.)
STRETCH-OUT (5 min.)	**Head Circles** **Shoulder Shrug** **Pike Body Stretch**	

W.E.T. PROGRESSIVE WORKOUT
Week 11

Vary the intensity of your W.E.T. set with "Fartlek" training: work for 30 seconds easy, then 30 seconds hard, then 30 seconds moderate. Repeat each W.E.T. in this manner.

WARM-UP (5 min.)	**Breathing and Bobbing** **Shoulder Shrug** **with "Chicken Wings"** **Log Roll**

W.E.T. Set
(20 min.)
	Upper: Rear Push-ups
	      Arm and Wrist Swirls
	      Reverse Scull
	
	SHAKE OUT
	
	Middle: Leg Swing
	      Hip Touch
	      Body Wave
	
	SHAKE OUT
	
	Lower: Leg Treading
	      Aqua-jog
	      Leg Crossover
	
	SHAKE OUT
	
	Combination: The Breaststroker
	          Treading
	          The Sidestroker

STRETCH-OUT (5 min.)	**Back Arch Stretch** **Static Ballet Leg Stretch** **Crossover Toe Touch**

W.E.T. PROGRESSIVE WORKOUT
Week 12

Add quantity to your quality. Now there are four W.E.T.s for each body area. Keep up your W.E.T. program to maintain your new-found fitness.

WARM-UP (5 min.)	Toe Tester Pike Body Stretch Breathing and Bobbing

W.E.T. SET
(20 min.)
	Upper: Sport Arm Pump
	    Water Push
	    Sport Swings and
	      Follow-Through

	SHAKE OUT

	Middle: Trunk Twist
	    Crab Stretch
	    Knee Tuck
	    Buttock Squeeze
	      with Crab Stretch

	SHAKE OUT

	Lower: Leg Lunge
	    Rockette Kick
	    Medley of Kicks
	    Disco Aqua Dancer

	SHAKE OUT

	Combination: The Backstroker
	    Ballet V
	    Coordinated Sport Arm
	    and Leg Motions
	    The Freestyler (with
	    breathing)

STRETCH-OUT
(5 min.)

Leg Split
Upward Bound
Static Arm Stretch

W.E.T. PROGRESSIVE WORKOUT
Week Lucky 13

It's up to you to keep maintaining your F.I.T.ness with your W.E.T. Workouts. Photocopy this page, and mix n' match to create your own W.E.T. Workout combinations! See chapter on "other" water horizons for additional suggestions.

W.E.T. PROGRESSIVE WORKOUT LOG

WARM-UP
(5 min.)

                                          *Time
and/or
Repetitions*

W.E.T. SET   **Upper:** _____   _____
(__ min.)

                                              SHAKE OUT

         Middle: _____   _____

SHAKE OUT

Lower: _____   _____

_____   _____

_____   _____

SHAKE OUT

Combination: _____   _____

_____   _____

_____   _____

STRETCH-OUT
(5 min.)

_____

_____

Part III

EXPAND YOUR
W.E.T. WORKOUTS

Add new dimensions to your W.E.T. Workouts by inviting friends and family members to join the W.E.T. set. The following are other suggested water activities.

Chapter 10

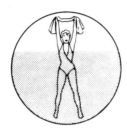

Spa W.E.T.s

Along with regular swimming pools, many health clubs and "Y's" offer water amenities known variously as whirlpools, spas, and hot tubs. Here, terms will be used interchangeably.

The following spa stretches are to help relax the body. These exercises can be used not only for general well-being, but also to help certain ailments, such as arthritis, fatigue tensions, and/or limited range of motion. They are isometric or static in nature (two forces pressing against each other—hold the stretched position for 30 seconds). Your total spa time should be no longer than 15 minutes. Remember to hold the stretch for 30 seconds; rest for 30 seconds so as not to overheat. Use the jets for intensified water-massaging action on various body parts such as ankle, knee, shoulder and wrist joints, and back.

FOOTSIES

Starting Position: Sit on the edge of the whirlpool with your feet just at the water's surface.

Technique: Rotate the lower legs so that your feet turn:

- inward
- outward
- forward and backward (up and down)
- sideways

Variations: Mix and match your rotations—try the eggbeater, which is realy an alternating Karate Kick.

SIT 'N' KICK

Starting Position: Sit at the edge of the whirlpool.

Technique: Begin with a slow rhythmic flutter kick—alternate kicks, e.g., dolphin (loose), breaststroke (flex feet as much as possible), etc. Concentrate on kicking slowly and try to keep your ankles flexible.

Variations: Change the intensity and speed of the kicks: 30 seconds of easy kicking; 30 seconds of rest; 30 seconds of moderate kicking; 30 seconds of rest.

146

Sit 'n' kick

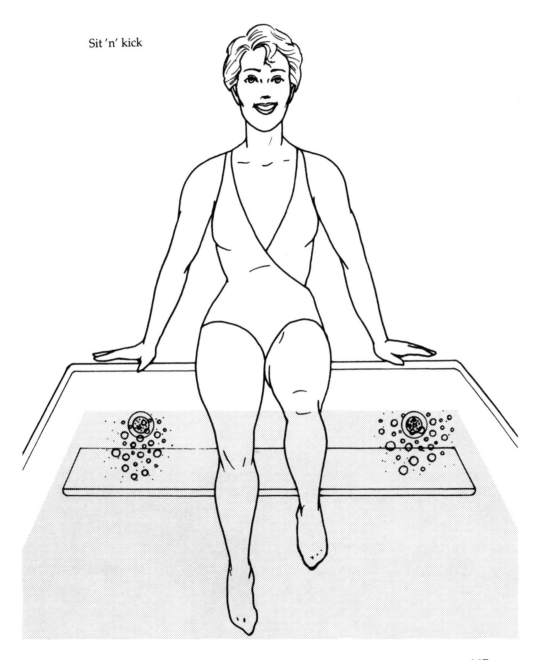

INDIAN SIT 'N' STRETCH

Starting Position: Sit in the bent-knee position, soles of the feet together.

Technique: Press your knees toward the bottom, stretching the inner thigh.

Variations: Rock from side to side.

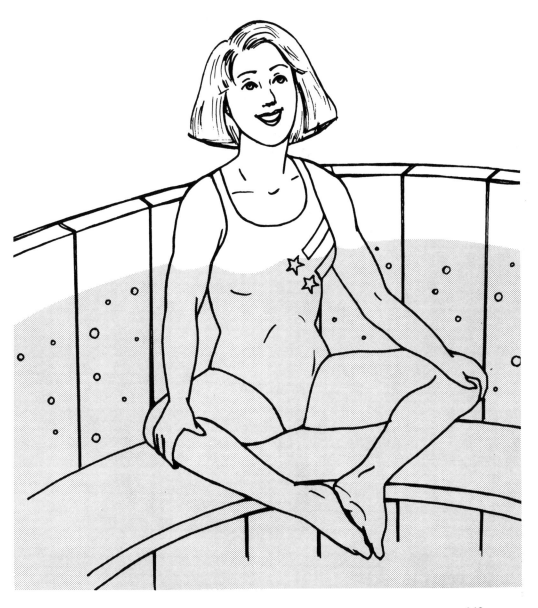

"V" VICTORY STRETCH

Starting Position: Sit in the corner of the tub with your back against the wall and your legs in a "V" position, the knees straight.

Technique: Separate your legs as far as possible, trying to touch the wall with your legs in the "V" position. Keep your legs straight and bring them together slowly, alternately crossing one leg over the other.

Variations: Alternately tilt your hips in the "V" position.

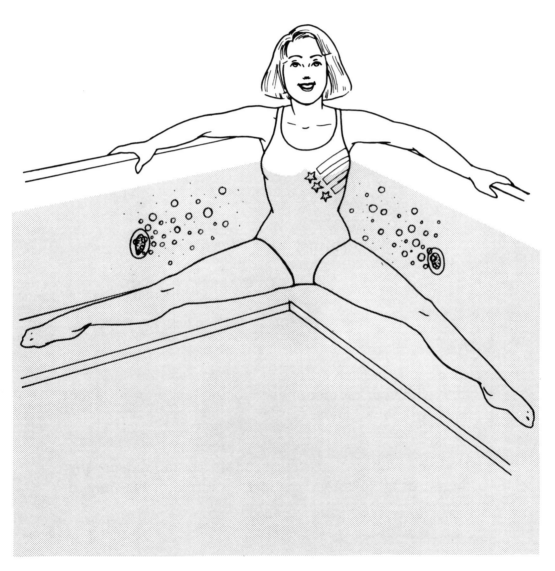

Chapter 11

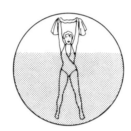

Partner, Family, Beach, and Home W.E.T.s

Doubling Your Pleasures

The following are water activities to be done with one or more partners.

- *Tub*

    Do a "tub" (a back float with bent knees in the tuck position) with your partner hooked foot to foot or head to foot. Scull with both hands.

- *Log Roll*

    Hook up with your partner head to foot in tandem. Then do a turn by pressing shoulders, and roll in the same direction.

- *Leap Frog*

    In chest-deep water, one person bends forward while the

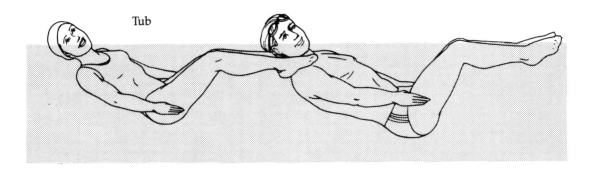

Tub

partner jumps over by placing his or her hands on the other's shoulders.

- *Two-Person Crawl Stroke*

  The leader does the crawl arm motion while the partner grasps his or her ankles with extended arms and does a flutter kick. Raise your head to breathe without pressing your partner's legs down. How far can you travel? How many different strokes can you combine? Try rolling over for the backstroke.

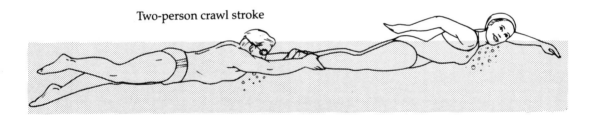

Two-person crawl stroke

- *Hi Jump*

  From a crouched position in chest-deep water, jump as high as possible. Try to out-jump your partner. You can also push off the wall and compare your glide distance to your partner's.

Partner Water Activities

Synchronize Your Strokes

Swim beside your partner and synchronize your arm strokes.

Underwater Charades

Imitate some action underwater and have your partner try to guess what you're doing. (Play cards, e.g.)

Jane and Tarzan

Try some ballet lifts in chest-deep water.

Join the W.E.T. Crowd

Remember, the more the better! Invite your family and friends to join you in W.E.T. Workouts.

Family Fun

The following are examples of water activities that can be done with your family members.

Introducing your little one to the water can be a good exercise, and it can be a great deal of fun, too. Play "motor boat" or train and engineer—here, you're going to pull your little one through the water and encourage him/her to kick and just let them enjoy the water, and always maintain eye contact with your child.

To help get your child go underwater, pretend it is his/her birthday and their cake is waterproof and it is under the water.

154

Have them "blow out" (exhale) all of the candles under the water.

For the family with four or more people, play a version of "Ring Around the Rosy." Here, you can practice submerging and going down to form bubbles. If there are a lot of people in the pool, play a "ball game" such as: water polo, water volleyball, water basketball (try a water hoop), or a simple game of catch with a light beach ball. These games are fun for both youngsters and for the young at heart. These games will get everyone going by involving everyone.

Water, Water Everywhere . . . Open-Water and Beach Activities

Sand Jog

Jog in calf-deep water at the beach. The deeper the water, the more energetic.

Crabwalk

Sitting at the water's edge, place your hands next to your hips. "Walk" forward, backward, sideways allowing legs to drag. For variation, do the crabwalk in the push-up position. The more of your body in the water, the easier it will be.

Sandy Sit-ups

At the water's edge, bury your feet in the sand, bend your knees, sit up and touch one of your elbows to the opposite knee. Repeat with the other elbow.

Leg Sand Sweeps

At the water's edge, press from an extended leg position and create sand circles by bringing your feet together and separating them.

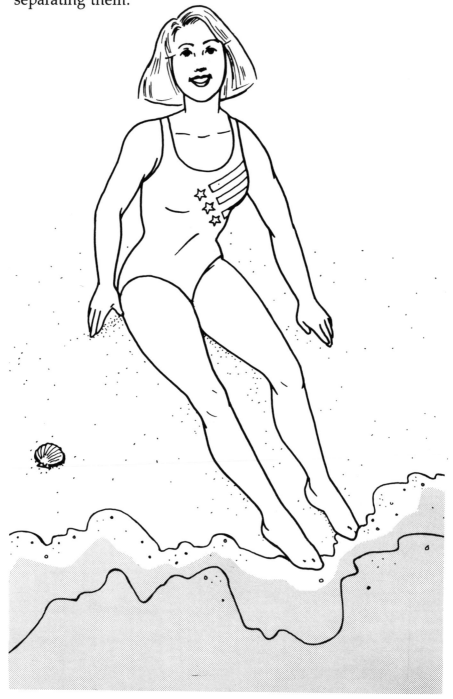

Surfer's Arm Paddle

From a balanced prone (face down) position on a raft or surf board, propel yourself using alternating forward arm circles (crawl stroke) or (simultaneously) a butterfly stroke.

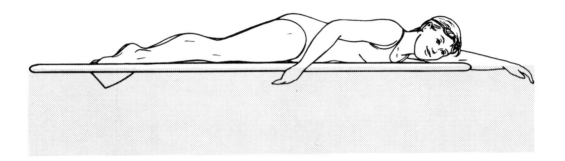

Home-Sweet-Home Water Activities

In your own bathtub (or someone else's!) do static arm and leg stretches, shoulder shrugs, breathing, buttock squeezes, foot, ankle, and wrist circles. Try an Indian Sit in the bathtub.

Isometric exercises can also be done in a tub. An isometric exercise is a contraction of the muscles in which the length of the muscle does not change. Here, you'll use your muscles to push or pull against an immovable object—the bathtub wall.

Press your hands against the inside of the tub wall in a sitting position. Hold for a maximum of 30 seconds and relax. Here your breath is held during your isometric exercise. Breathe deeply between contractions.

Depending on the size of your tub (and you), try an isometric leg press with your feet pressing against the front of the tub. Hold for a maximum of 30 seconds and relax.

You can also practice your breathing in several inches of lukewarm water, right in the privacy of your own sink.

Practice rhythmic breathing at home.

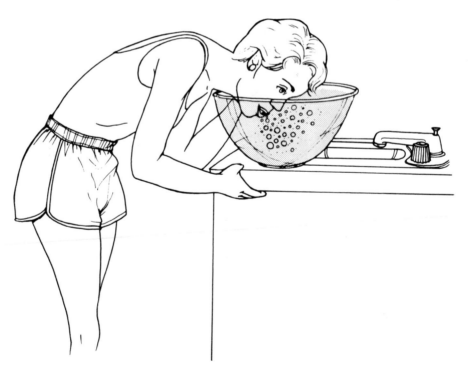

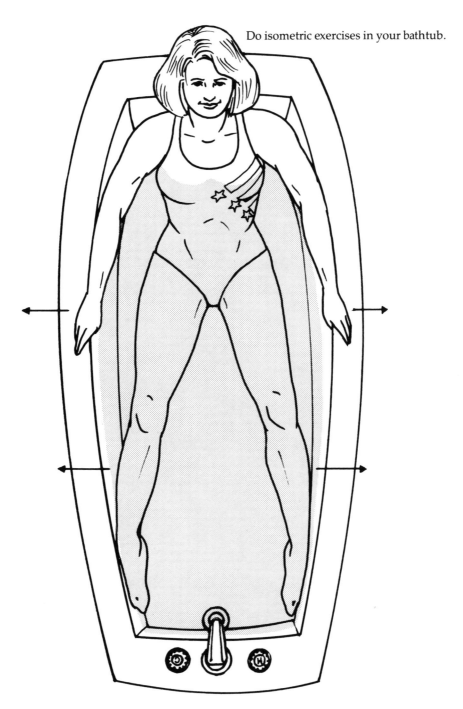

Do isometric exercises in your bathtub.

Part IV

Q's AND A's
FOR YOUR W.E.T.s

Getting Started and Keeping at It

Q. *Am I too old to start an exercise program?*

A. You're never too old to start an exercise program. However, if you have not been physically active, I strongly urge you to get a physical examination and a stress test especially if you're over age 35. If your physician says you're in good shape to begin an exercise program, then by all means, get started. Generally speaking, water exercise is probably the best all-around activity for somebody who is starting out on the road to physical fitness. Certainly it is not as strenuous or bone jarring as jogging. Many over-40's are out there exercising, and they are doing amazing things; so, age should not be a barrier to starting a program of physical fitness.

Remember the unique benefits of water: buoyancy (you only weigh 10% of your body weight in water), relaxa-

tion, increased range of motion, aerobic exercise benefits—and most of all, it's refreshing and fun!

Q. *Will I experience any discomfort doing W.E.T.s?*

A. You should feel that you have had a rewarding workout;
however, if you experience any serious discomfort during
your workout, stop and rest, then continue. If the discomfort continues, your body is trying to tell you that
something is not right, and you must stop and see your
doctor. Always listen to your body.

Q. *My muscles are too tight; will I be able to use W.E.T.s?*

A. Yes, but start with the relaxed version of the exercises.
As you progress, your muscles will become more supple
and the exercises will become easier for you.

Q. *Why do I feel stiff and sore after a W.E.T. Workout, and what
can I do about it?*

A. You may experience some discomfort at the start of your
W.E.T. program because you're using muscles that have
been inactive. Be certain to warm up properly. You may
wish to switch to the relaxed version of specific W.E.T.s.
If pain or discomfort persists, consult your doctor.

Q. *Why do I get cramps and what can I do about them?*

A. A cramp is a contraction, or tightening, of the muscle
fibers. It is usually caused by lack of a warm-up or by
overexertion. There is a warning sign; you feel tension in
the area, usually the leg. This should be your signal to
stop or ease up. Listen to your body.

   If a cramp does occur, apply direct pressure to the area
by squeezing and pressing the affected muscle deeply
with your thumbs. Rest before continuing your W.E.T.s.

Q. *What should I do when I feel discouraged about my progress?*

A. Don't give up. The road to physical fitness is never short, and it requires dedication and self-discipline to reach your goals. So when you hit the doldrums, just remind yourself that at the end of the road there will be a healthier and happier you. Hang in there and go for it!

Q. *I'm so busy during the week that I really don't have the time to exercise—I can only exercise on the weekends. What can I do about this?*

A. Get your long exercise sessions in on the weekends, and try to supplement these with shorter sessions during the week—try to exercise at least twice during the week. Remember there are 24 hours in each day, and, after sleep and work, you should have at least eight hours left. Schedule one hour for exercise—no matter what, you should try to get that one hour for yourself. Discuss this with your family, associates, and friends; if they see you are determined to get fit, I am sure they will support your efforts—and who knows, you may involve some of them.

Q. *How much time should I devote to a W.E.T. routine?*

A. Ideally, do your W.E.T.s 3 times per week. Begin with a 20-minute workout, including a 5-minute warm-up, a 10-minute W.E.T. set, and a 5-minute cool-down.

Q. *Why do I feel tired after exercising?*

A. Your aerobic capacity is developing and improving, and if you have not been exercising regularly, you may feel tired. Start with the relaxed variation and try to follow the program for at least three times a week. Exercising regularly will ultimately give you more energy. Stay with it!

Q. *Can I do W.E.T. Workouts during my menstrual period?*

A. There is no reason why you should not. If you experience discomfort, you may be more comfortable doing the "relaxed" level of your W.E.T.s.

Balancing Your Diet With W.E.T.s

Q. *If I go on a weight reducing diet, why do I have to exercise?*

A. Dieting alone may help you lose excess weight, but diet and exercise together will help you reach your ideal weight much more quickly. Also, dieting alone will not firm up your muscles and improve your shape, only exercise can do that. Many dieters are disappointed because they frequently regain their lost weight, but a consistent exercise program can help break that cycle and keep you at your ideal weight.

Q. *As long as I am exercising, do I have to worry about my diet?*

A. Exercise alone will not use up enough calories to help you lose weight unless you are going to exercise for two to three hours a day—which, for most of us, is not possible. Diet and exercise should always go hand in hand.

Q. *How many calories should I consume to lose weight or maintain a desired weight?*

A. This depends on several factors—age, activity level, health, individual metabolism, etc. However, if you're over 21, approximate your required caloric intake by multiplying your desired weight by 15. For example, if you want to maintain a body weight of 120 pounds, your daily caloric intake would be about 1,800 calories (120 × 15 = 1,800). Keep in mind that if you are physically active, your daily caloric intake should not drop below 1,200. Remember that exercise and dieting go hand in hand in weight reduction.

Q. *How can I calculate weight loss?*

A. There are 3,500 calories per pound of body weight. If you eat 500 fewer calories a day and maintain the same activity level, you would start to lose weight. If you used up 3,500 calories per week your net weight loss for the year would be about 50 pounds. After your W.E.T.s your metabolism is increased, which helps to burn more calories.

Q. *If I exercise, should I increase my intake of protein?*

A. Not necessarily. Your body uses carbohydrates for its fuel, and you should eat more of these, but in the form of fresh fruits and vegetables, grains and grain products. Be sure you eat a balanced diet that provides you with the required vitamins and minerals. Try to drink at least eight glasses of water a day, to replace the water you lose through perspiration.

Q. *I've heard that exercise acts as an appetite suppressant. How does it do this?*

A. As you exercise, the blood that is not needed in your stomach and intestines is shunted to your heart, lungs, and muscles where it *is* needed. After your exercise session, research has shown, it may take up to three or four hours for the blood to return to your stomach, and until the blood returns to your stomach, your body cannot digest food very well; therefore, you often do not feel the need to eat. This is your body's way of telling you to wait before you eat.

You're Beautiful—With W.E.T.s

Q. *What kind of bathing suit is best for doing my W.E.T. Workouts?*

A. Choose a bathing suit that is comfortable, lightweight, and becoming to your body. Be certain that there are no uncomfortable string or strap placements that can rise up or slip down and that your buttocks and bust are secure. Lycra is comfortable, and one size does fit most people; however, check the life of your suit if you use it often—lycra suits will eventually develop threadbare areas at the hips, bust, or buttocks. The life of a nylon suit is longer, but many people find them less comfortable. There are also various combination fabrics available on the market. Whatever your suit is made of, be sure to rinse it thoroughly after each use to prolong its life.

Q. *Is chlorine harmful?*

A. Chlorine is used in pools to keep them free of bacteria and algae. It won't hurt you. However, the combination of chlorine and water can dry your skin and hair.

Q. *What can I do to protect my skin?*

A. Use your favorite moisturizer just after your W.E.T. Workout. Shower as usual, and apply your moisturizer to moist skin to help replace the natural oils that have been depleted by the water.

Q. *Can I protect my skin from the sun's rays while doing my W.E.T. workouts at the beach?*

A. Yes, use a waterproof sunscreen with PABA and a high sun protection factor. After your W.E.T. Workout, reapply the sunscreen because it will wear off after a period of time because of perspiration and water.

Q. *What can I do to protect my hair?*

A. If you need to keep your hair dry, choose W.E.T. Workouts that keep your chin above water. Also use a sweatband around your hairline to help protect it against any surprise splashes. You can protect your hair with a bathing cap, too. For extra protection, apply your favorite conditioner to your hair tips. Remember to shower after each W.E.T. Workout and apply a hair conditioner or creme rinse.

Q. *Should I wear goggles while doing my W.E.T. Workouts?*

A. Most of your W.E.T. Workouts can be done without submerging your face. However, if you wear contact lenses and/or you are combining your W.E.T. Workouts with swimming, goggles are recommended. (Prescription goggles are available.)

Q. *How can I protect my ears during W.E.T. Workouts?*

A. Many of the W.E.T.s are done with your head above water. If you wish to prevent water from entering the ear canal, I suggest the following:

- EAR PLUGS: These seal your outer ear canal; they are reasonably priced and easily available.

- LAMB'S WOOL: (available in drugstores and swim stores) Place a small piece of lamb's wool into your outer ear canal and seal it with petroleum jelly.

- BATHING CAP: Use a snug-fitting bathing cap that covers your ears.

Q. *Do I need nose clips?*

A. If you feel uncomfortable exhaling through your nose while submerging, nose clips will help. However, practice exhaling through your nose while bobbing. Soon it will become more comfortable, and you may not need nose clips.

Q. *How can I protect my nails in the water?*

A. You can help protect the life and luster of your nails with buffing as well as various nail hardeners and protective coatings on the market. You can seal your nails by coating the exposed underside of each nail with a pre-coat polish, nail conditioner, or hardener.

Spas and Safety

Q. *What are the unique benefits of using a spa?*

A. Besides the other benefits of water, spas add the following advantage: The spa jets massage the body. Massage is known to promote healing of injuries by increasing blood circulation, which increases the oxygen and waste product exchange in the body tissues. This allows the by-products of inflammation to be removed more quickly. In addition, the pressure of the water massage helps reduce swelling.

Q. *What safety precautions should you be aware of when using a spa?*

A. Read the signs posted at the spa. If you have an illness or a health condition such as pregnancy, do not use the spa. Also, with the foaming water you may not see a step or may lose your balance. In rare cases, bacterial infections can be contracted from sitting on bench areas close to spas.

Q. *How long should I stay in a spa or hot tub?*

A. If the water temperature is 104° F (40° C) do not remain in the tub for longer than 15 minutes.

Q. *Why such a short time?*

A. High water temperatures can raise the body's temperature and the temperature of your internal organs beyond safe limits—it would be similar to having a fever. If you wish to remain in the spa for longer than 15 minutes, you may:
1. lower the temperature of the water to body temperature, 98.6°F, or
2. leave the spa after 15 minutes, take a shower, cool down, and return.

Q. *Can I do exercises in a spa?*

A. Yes, a spa is ideal for doing warm-ups; you can do some simple stretches. However, don't overdo it, and don't stay in the spa for longer than 15 minutes.

Q. *Can young children use a spa or hot tub?*

A. Yes, but they need supervision, and they need instruction on how to enter and how to leave the spa or hot tub. They should know that spas and hot tubs are not made for jumping, diving, or for swimming underwater. Never let kids use the spa unsupervised. For children, the temperature of the water in the spa or hot tub should be close to body temperature.

Q. *What safety precautions should I be aware of around water?*

A. In a pool, look before you plunge! Check for water clarity, depth, other bathers, safety equipment, diving boards, and for lifeguards on duty. Remember: Never swim alone.

In open-water area, check for posted precautions, including water temperature, currents, tides, submerged pilings, etc. Never dive into unknown waters. Learn artificial respiration (AR) and cardiopulmonary resuscitation (CPR) by taking a course offered by your local American Red Cross or American Heart Associaton chapter.

Q. *Does swimming pool water make you more susceptible to infections?*

A. Pool water is chemically treated and filtered continuously for your safety and comfort. The key to keeping your body less susceptible to infection is to dry off properly after your workout. (There is always a fungus among us!) If you are susceptible to athlete's foot or jock itch, be certain to dry these areas thoroughly, and use a powder or cream made for either of these problems. Women will find that water does not enter the vagina because of the overlapping of the anterior and posterior walls. Be certain before you plunge into the pool, to check the odor, clarity, and cleanliness of the water. If the pool has a chronic "ring around the collar," you may want to look for another facility.

Q. *After my W.E.T. Workouts, I get thirsty. What should I drink?*

A. Water! It is an essential nutrient with zero calories that will replenish your internal water supply after exercise. It's best to drink cool water, which will enter the bloodstream at a faster rate; and remember, even though you're in water and so can't see any sweat, you *are* perspiring. So replenish your vital water supply with H_2O.

R$_x$ and W.E.T. Workouts

Q. *I've recently recovered from a bone fracture. When can I do W.E.T.s?*

A. As soon as you get your Rx from your doctor to start bearing weight again. Begin your W.E.T.s slowly. Use the relaxed variations of your W.E.T.s and then move to more difficult levels. Do not overdo it; progress slowly and comfortably.

Q. *I'm a dancer who's plagued by leg injuries. Can W.E.T. Workouts be helpful to me?*

A. You have already overstretched your leg muscles; rather than overemphasize stretching, focus on coordinating, strengthening, and the aerobic qualities of W.E.T. Workouts.

Q. *I'm a weekend athlete plagued by injuries. Can W.E.T. Workouts help my aches and pains?*

A. If your particular sport movement hurts out of water, simulate your sport swing with your upper-body W.E.T. Workouts (relaxed variation) to the point of comfort (not pressure or pain). As healing occurs, the faster and more energetically you can exercise against the water's resistance and the more strength you'll obtain.

Q. *I have a chronic back (knee, shoulder, etc.) condition; can W.E.T. Workouts help?*

A. Choose the W.E.T. Workouts that are comfortable for you. Remember that the massaging effect of water, especially

173

the forceful jet of a whirlpool or spa, helps to increase circulation in the area. Place the affected area in front of the jet.

Q. *Can W.E.T. Workouts help me relax after my tennis match, round of golf, etc.?*

A. Yes, the massaging and relaxing effects of the water (especially warm water) will help ease those land-made aches and pains.

Q. *I have a heart condition; are W.E.T. Workouts good for me?*

A. When you get your doctor's okay to exercise, begin your W.E.T. Workouts slowly and do the relaxed version. W.E.T. Workouts are a good alternative to terra-firma activities, even if you are not a swimmer.

Gear Up for W.E.T.s at the Source

Q. *What are some of the different types of swim gear and what are they used for?*

A. The most common types of swim gear are:
FINS—these are used to add variety to your workouts; they help develop the muscles in your thighs, calves, and abdomen; the resistance placed on these muscles helps both to improve your cardiovascular capacity and to make your feet and ankles more flexible. Fins come in men's and women's sizes, and the shoe-type is the kind I recommend.
PULL-BUOYS—these are two cylinders made of Styrofoam held together by two cords or straps. They come in various sizes and the larger the buoy, the more buoyancy it

provides. The pull-buoy supports your legs so you can work on your arm strokes. It is used primarily when you want to learn a new stroke, improve technique, and to build upper-body strength.

FLOATS—these are small inflatable cuffs that are fitted around your arms or ankles or both. They provide both buoyancy and resistance during a workout.

HAND PADDLES—these are plastic plates that fit over your palms and act like fins for your hands. They are resistance devices, and they strengthen your shoulders, chest, arm, and back muscles. They are also used to help you improve your swimming form.

TUBES—these are small rubber devices that are twisted in a figure "8" around your ankles. They are used to create more drag so you can build up more power in your stroke.

OTHER DEVICES—Among these are wrist and ankle weights, drag suits and vests, and kickboards with scooped-out bottoms. All of these are used to improve total body conditioning.

Q. *Where can I find the latest swim gear?*

A. Begin looking in your local swim shop, large department stores, and sporting goods store. Use the Yellow Pages to find the nearest location. Most of these stores will usually carry general swim gear, including swimsuits, caps, goggles, nose clips, ear plugs, and arm flotation devices. For standard and specialty swim gear, write or call the suppliers in the following list:

Adidas
c/o LIBCO
1 Silver Court
Springfield, NJ 07081
(201) 379-1630

AMF/HEAD Sportswear, Inc.
9189 Red Branch Road
Columbia, MD 21045
(301) 730-8300
In Canada:

175

225 Chabanel Street West
Montreal, PQ

Arena U.S.A. Inc.
23880 Hawthorne Blvd.
Torrance, CA 90505
(213) 373-7767

Competitive Aquatic Supply
Division of Modern Swim
   Concepts
P.O. Box K
4128-A South Street
Lakewood, CA 90714
(213) 633-3333

Danskin, Inc.
1114 Avenue of the Americas
New York, NY 10036
(212) 869-9800

The Finals
Division of Ardmore
149 Mercer Street
New York, NY 10012
(212) 431-1414
NY/NJ—call collect
Toll-free number: 800-221-8550

Hind-Wells, Inc.
390 Buckley Road
San Luis Obispo, CA 93401
(805) 544-8555
Toll-free number outside
   California: 800-235-4150

Jantzen, Inc.
P.O. Box 3001
Portland, OR 97208
(503) 238-5000

National Aquatic Service
1425 Erie Boulevard East
Syracuse, N.Y. 13210

(315) 479-5544—call collect in
   New York State
Toll-free number: 800-448-5521
   outside New York State

Ocean Pool Supply Co., Inc.
Stepar Place
Huntington Station, L.I., N.Y.
   11746
(516) 427-5200

Rothhammer International, Inc.
P.O. Box 2959
Lancaster, CA 93539
(805) 943-5129

Speedo of America, Inc.
380 S.E. Spokane St.
Portland, OR 97222
Toll-free number, Western U.S.:
   800-547-4601
Toll-free number, Eastern U.S.:
   800-547-4687

Sunwear Corporation
330 Fifth Avenue
New York, N.Y. 10001
(212) 563-5595

The Swim Shop
1400 Eighth Avenue South
P.O. Box 1402
Nashville, TN 37203
Toll-free number: 800-251-1412

Uglies Unlimited
1617 E. Highland
Phoenix, AZ 85016
Toll-free number: 800-528-3650

World Wide Aquatics
509 Wyoming Avenue
Cincinnati, OH 45215
Toll-free number: 800-543-4459

This is by no means an exhaustive list, but you should be able to find all the swim gear you will need from these companies.

In addition to the preceding companies, you can contact the following for more complete aquatic information.

American National Red Cross
Seventeenth and D Streets, N.W.
Washington, D.C. 20006
(202) 737-8300

International Swimming Hall of
   Fame
1 Hall of Fame Drive
Fort Lauderdale, FL 33316
(305) 462-6536

National Jewish Welfare Board
15 East 26th Street
New York, NY 10010
(212) 532-4949

National Spa and Pool Institute
2111 Eisenhower Avenue
Alexandria, VA 22314
(703) 838-0083

"Y"s of U.S.A.
101 N. Wacker Drive
Chicago, IL 60606
(312) 977-0031

Information for aquatics
   programs and materials at local
   chapters.

National Aquatic Museum
   equipment, etc.

Information about local aquatic
   programs at YM-YWHA's and
   Jewish community centers.

National trade association for
   pool and spa manufacturers

Comprehensive programs in local
   YM & YWCA's throughout
   country

For the Complete W.E.T. Enthusiast

Q. *What gear whould I keep in my locker or swim bag?*

A. I suggest that you have the following:

bathing suit	lamb's wool
bathing cap	petroleum jelly
goggles	eye and ear drops (in case of
waterproof watch	irritation)

sweatband
towel
sunscreen (if you're swimming
   outdoors)
hair clip and hair bands
hair shampoo and conditioner
razor
shaving cream
face and body moisturizer
astringent
body powder
cotton swabs—to clean ears;
   apply makeup
cotton balls—for makeup removal
hairbrush and comb
hair dryer (if not provided by the
   pool facility)

body cologne
nail polish and nail amenities
eye and lip makeup—waterproof
   brands if for swimming
   purposes
plastic bags—for wet bathing
   suits
small box—for telephone change
plastic pouch—to keep jewelry,
   contact lens paraphernalia
business cards and pen because
   "you never know who you're
   going to meet."
a compartmentalized plastic box
   or basket—to organize your
   locker

See you poolside!

Index

Index